CARDIAC SURGERY - A COMMITMENT TO SCIENCE, TECHNOLOGY AND CREATIVITY

Edited by **Miguel Angel Maluf and Paulo Roberto Barbosa Évora**

Cardiac Surgery - A Commitment to Science, Technology and Creativity
http://dx.doi.org/10.5772/50590
Edited by Miguel Angel Maluf and Paulo Roberto Barbosa Évora

Contributors

Miguel Angel Maluf, Paulo Roberto B. Evora, Gilberto Barbosa, Francisco Gregory, Glauco Glauco Lobo, Luis Alberto Oliveira Dallan, Nina Vinicius José, Renato S. Assad

Published by InTech

Janeza Trdine 9, 51000 Rijeka, Croatia

Publishing Process Manager Sandra Bakic
Technical Editor InTech DTP team
Cover InTech Design team

First published February, 2014
Printed in Croatia

Additional hard copies can be obtained from orders@intechopen.com

Cardiac Surgery - A Commitment to Science, Technology and Creativity, Edited by Miguel Angel Maluf and Paulo Roberto Barbosa Évora
p. cm.
ISBN 978-953-51-1228-0

For EU product safety concerns:
IN TECH d.o.o., Prolaz Marije Krucifikse Kozulić 3, 51000 Rijeka, Croatia,
info@intechopen.com or visit our website at intechopen.com.

Meet the editors

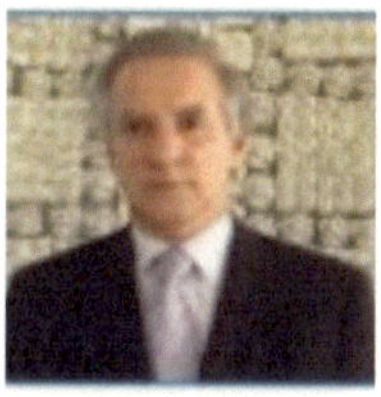

Dr. Miguel Angel Maluf was born in Córdoba, Argentina in 1950. He has graduated from Universidade Nacional de Córdoba, Argentina and become a medical doctor in 1973. Dr. Maluf did specalization in Cardiovascular Surgery at Instituto do Coracao (INCOR) – São Paulo, Brazil. His Surgical Fellowship training was finished by defending the Master's, Dosctoral and Postdoctoral thesis, in the Cardiovascular Division at Universidade Federal de São Paulo, Brazil. He research includes development of several models of biological cardiac prosthetic to remodeling of the right ventricle outlet tract, in congential heart disease. Dr. Maluf has more than 25 internattional plus 40 national publications, as well as 80 international and 250 national presentations and more then 11 book chapters related to his research areas. Currently he works as Associate Professor of the Cardiovascular Division at São Paulo Federal University.

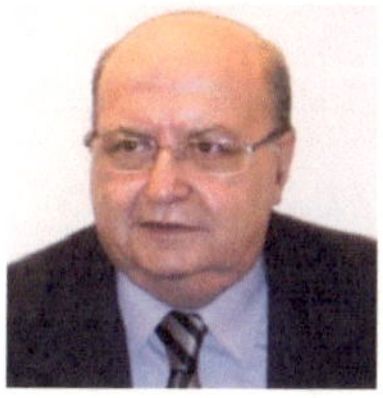

Paulo Roberto Barbosa Evora graduated in Medicine at the Ribeirão Preto School of Medicine,University of São Paulo, SP, Brazil (1972); medical resident in General Surgery (1973) and Thoracic and Cardiovascular Surgery (1974), obtaining the doctor's degree (1980) in General Surgery at the Postgraduate Program of the Department of Surgery and Anatomy. Dr. Evora participated in the Post- Doctoral and Visiting Researcher in Cardiovascular Surgical Research (1990-1991) and as Senior Research Fellow in Research Surgery (1991-192) at the Mayo Graduate School of Medicine, Mayo Foundation, Rochester, USA. He became an Associate Professor in Thoracic and Cardiovascular Surgery at the Department of Surgery and Anatomy, Ribeirão Preto Faculty of Medicine, University of São Paulo in 1993. Exerted all his academic work as Assistant Physician at Ribeirão Preto Hospital of Clinics , where he served as Clinical Director of Intensive Care during 27 years at the end of 2003 he started obtaining the position of professor in Public Defense (2004), held the position of Coordinator of the Endothelial Function of the Division of Experimental Surgery. His current research includes following topics : 1) Global ischemia and reperfusion; 2)Vasoplegic endothelial dysfunction; 3) Effects of mechanical forces on the vasoreactivity of human saphenous veins, and; 4) Acid-base balance and endothelium-dependent vascular reactivity.

Contents

Preface IX

Chapter 1 **New Polyurethane Prostheses for Substitution of Cardiac Valve Disease and Remodeling of the Right Ventricle in Congenital Heart Malformations 1**
Miguel A. Maluf, Hector A. Barone and Fabricio Sena

Chapter 2 **Adult Cardiopulmonary Bypass in the Twenty-First Century — Science, Art or Empiricism? 11**
Paulo Roberto Barbosa Evora and Alfredo José Rodrigues

Chapter 3 **Hands on as Educational Process in Cardiovascular Surgery 35**
Gilberto Venossi Barbosa, Carlos Manuel de Almeida Brandão and Vinicius José da Silva Nina

Chapter 4 **Conservative Management of Mitral Insufficiency — An Alternative Approach 59**
Francisco Gregori Junior

Chapter 5 **Coronary Artery Bypass Grafting Without Cardiopulmonary Bypass and Without Aortic Manipulation 71**
José Glauco Lobo Filho, Heraldo Guedis Lobo Filho and Eduardo Rebouças Carvalho

Chapter 6 **Use of Inhaled Nitric Oxide in Cardiac Surgery: What is Going on? 85**
Alfredo José Rodrigues, Patricia Martinez Evora and Paulo Roberto Barbosa Evora

Chapter 7 **Mechanical Complications of Acute Myocardial Infarction 101**
Luís Augusto Palma Dallan, Luiz Roberto Palma Dallan, Luiz Augusto Ferreira Lisboa and Luís Alberto Oliveira Dallan

Chapter 8 **Hypoplastic Left Heart Syndrome: Why Use a Hybrid Procedure? 115**
Miguel Maluf

Chapter 9 **Surgical Repair of Stenotic Pulmonary Arteries in Tetralogy of Falllot 125**
Vinicius José da Silva Nina

Chapter 10 **Adjustable Pulmonary Artery Banding 149**
Renato S. Assad

Preface

It is a great pleasure for me to be the editor of this book. Nowadays, there is lot of classical adult and pediatric cardiac surgery text books describing various well-known topics. This book is composed of chapters with reference to issues of today. The authors of these chapters are recognized heart surgeons with renowned training in centers of the U.S. and Europe.

In this book it is shown how this specialty has evolved over the past 20 years, with significant advances in diagnosis and palliative and definitive techniques for correction of cardiovascular diseases. These changes in posture against congenital or acquired heart disease has stimulated the cooperative work of Cardiologists and Cardiac Surgeons in training the Heart Team, now working in hybrid rooms to complement the more complex procedures. Procedures have been simplified, the results improved and patients benefited from it. Pediatric cardiology section enlightens us on cardiovascular changes in future infants as well. The search for new biomaterials such as polyurethane for the construction of heart valves, opens new possibilities especially for pediatric cardiac prosthesis. In conclusion; these 10 chapters are showing the classical adult and pediatric cardiac surgery .

At the end, I would like to thank all the contributors to this book, who spent part of their time in preparation of their chapters, showing alternative techniques which developed over the years .

Miguel Angel Maluf, MD, PhD
Cardiovascular Surgeon
Associate Professor
Cardiovascular Division
São Paulo Federal University
São Paulo – Brazil

Paulo Roberto Évora, MD, PhD
Cardiovascular Surgeon
Associate Professor
Cardiovascular Division
Riberão Preto Faculty
São Paulo University
São Paulo – Brazil

Chapter 1

New Polyurethane Prostheses for Substitution of Cardiac Valve Disease and Remodeling of the Right Ventricle in Congenital Heart Malformations

Miguel A. Maluf, Hector A. Barone and Fabricio Sena

Additional information is available at the end of the chapter

http://dx.doi.org/10.5772/57112

1. Introduction

The presence of an obstruction in the outflow tract of the right ventricle (RV) consists of a relatively common defect, present in 20% to 30% of cyanotic congenital heart diseases. The extreme degree of pulmonary obstruction is pulmonary atresia (anatomical discontinuity between RV - Pulmonary Artery), present in approximately 5% of patients with heart defects. In these situations, surgical treatment may require the use of a prosthesis or implantation of a valved conduit to reconstruct the pulmonary valve and outflow tract of the RV. Different valve replacements have been proposed, including the fresh aortic homografts, pulmonary heterografts, pig or bovine pericardial prostheses. Amongst the valved conduits we have: bovine pericardial grafts, porcine pulmonary graft, bovine jugular containing Dacron prostheses, aortic homograft, or more recently, pulmonary homografts. Mechanical prostheses were virtually abandoned. Whichever type of replacement valve used, many studies have reported calcification or tissue degeneration associated to pseudo-intimal proliferation and progressive obstruction of the conduit [1], [2], [3], [4], [5] with the need for reoperation, the incidence of which may vary between 14% and 30% at 5 years and 32% to 100% at 10 years. [4], [5], [6], [7], [8] In 1991, we began a new experience in the Cardiovascular Division of the Federal University of São Paulo (Unifesp), using 2 models of biological prostheses: heterografts (swine) treated with glutaraldehyde and formaldehyde [9], adding in recent years other 2 models. These 4 different prostheses were implanted in 203 children with heart defects that required reconstruction of the pulmonary valve and right ventricular outflow tract. [10] The late outcome of these patients is represented by actuarial Kaplan & Meier curve: The survival of these patients was 86.6% operated and free reoperations in 68.3% of cases, in 180 months of median rate of follow-up. (Figure 1) The most frequent cause of reoperations was calcification, tissue degeneration and loss of function due to growth of the patient.

The implantation of a bioprosthetic porcine valve in a patient, is considered as a form of living tissue transplantation. Xenotransplantation, which usually has a very aggressive form of rejection by the immune system of the patient. Aiming to reduce this type of immunogenicity, bioprostheses are fixed in glutaraldehyde solution, with the intention of transforming the tissue graft immunologically inert.

However, bioprostheses that were fixed in glutaraldehyde also have the propensity to calcify. This calcification is a major contributor for dysfunction of cardiac bioprostheses due to the pre-treatment of biological tissue with glutaraldehyde to devitalize the cells ceasing residual cells that become the primary sites for deposition of calcium phosphate. The reaction of calcium with the extracellular fluid associated with the reactions of phosphorus to the cell membrane causes pathological calcification of bioprostheses.

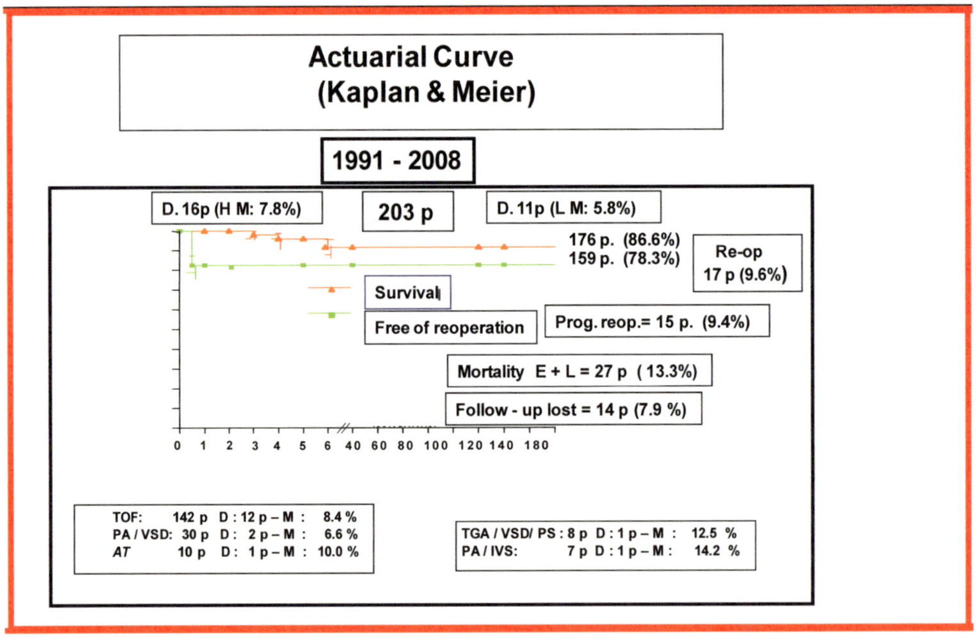

Figure 1. Actuarial curve of patients undergoing reconstruction of the pulmonary valve and outflow tract of the right ventricle with pulmonary heterograft. (Miguel Maluf, *The Heart Surgery Forum 2011; 14 (1): E40-50.*

Despite the deterioration of the heterograft keeps the order of 35% to 45% in 15 and 20 years, respectively. There are always isolated cases with long postoperative course, without compromising tissue or calcification of porcine bioprostheses. [11].

During the last decade there was an excellent immediate biocompatibility of *polycarbonourethane* valves *(PCU)* used in temporary ventricular assistance. [12] Although the follow-up in this group of patients is quite short, low rates of thromboembolic complications and no failures or calcification have been documented. Such valves were implanted experimentally, replacing heart valves and satisfactory results in long-term left ventricular assistance devices in between the apex of the left ventricle and the aorta. [13] Furthermore, the replacement valve is used in a next generation of total artificial heart implants. [14] However, the intermediate result of such artificial valves, when the prosthesis is implanted on the right side of the heart, exposed to low pressure and low levels of oxygen saturation, the prosthesis would have increased durability. The *segmented polyurethanes (SPUs)* are a class of versatile material possessing various controllable properties. This unique feature can make them advantageous for use as biomaterials, structural materials and other applications.

More than 50 years of research has been devoted to this area, which led to an understanding of the synthesis, structure and properties of these fascinating materials. In general, the *SPUs* have a structure comprising a *macrodiol* "soft" segment (SS) and *urethane* "hard" segment (SH), each segment has an incompatible composition with the separation of different phase driving nanoscale domains which control properties of *SPUs*. It is believed that HSS, glassy or crystalline, has the melting temperature (Tm) above room temperature. Forman domains are on the order of a few tens of nanometers. These domains SSs, are difficult to separate and are generally formed at low temperature to the glass transition (Tg) of amorphous to crystalline.

2. Objectives of research

The objectives of this study are:

To build a heart prosthesis of *segmented polyurethane (SPU)*

2.1. Methods

a. Drawing in 3D of a human aortic valve, obtained from an examination of Angio-Computerized Tomography (Angio-CT)

b. Matrix of the prosthesis.

c. Prepare of segmented polyurethane (SPU).

d. Manufacture of prosthesis by injection of SPU in the matrix.

2.2. Building a model of segmented *Polyurethane (SPU)* prosthesis

a. Design of the prosthesis in 3 D and Manufacturing of Moulds:

The 3-D drawing for manufacturing of the *polyurethane* was based on anatomical characteristics of Angio-CT of the human aortic and pulmonary valve.

We considered internal and external diameter, shape of the ring and stem where they operate the valve leaflets.

The valve leaflets were preserved, an angle of 120° from the place of central coaptation to the base of the valve ring deployment. Each leaflet has a thickness in the central region of the free edge of 0.2 mm and 0.5 mm in the rest of the extension. The program to be used for the design of this prosthesis is generated by Solid Works software, the computer program generates mesh and solid parametric.

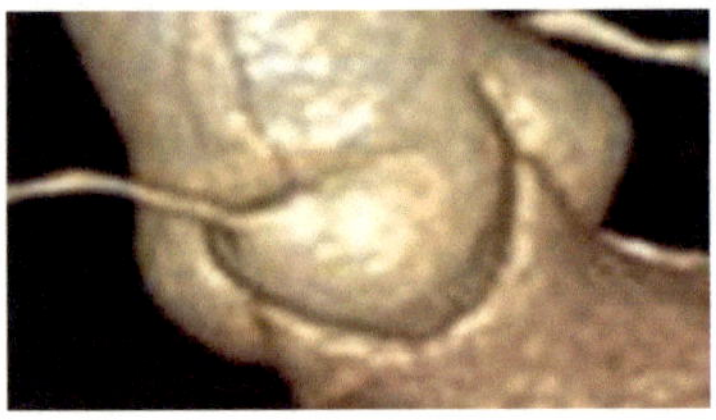

Figure 2. Angio Computerized Tomography (Angio-TC) of a human Aortic Valve

- Modeling of the Ring and Membrane

From pre-established dimensions by Angio-CT, the software was modeled using the ring and the membranes of the 3 cusps. figures 2,3,4

- Drawing of the Ring

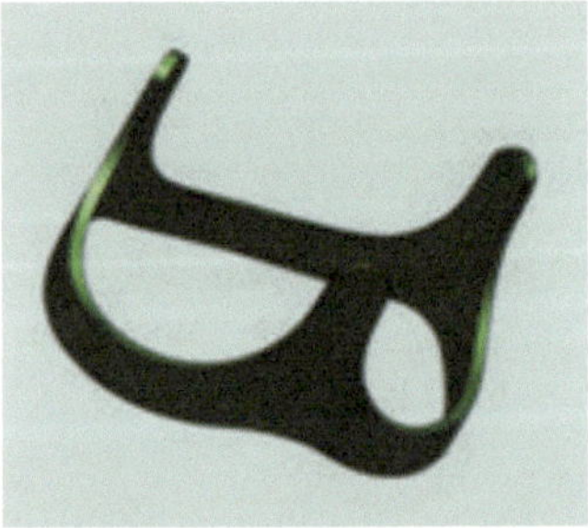

Figure 3. Drawing of a prosthetic ring

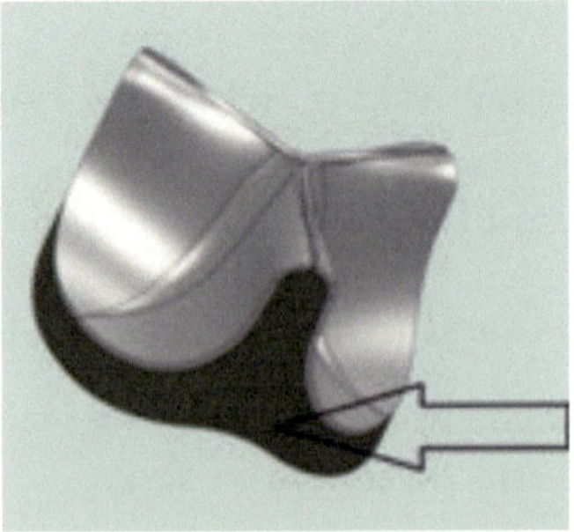

Figure 4. Drawing of three leaflets of the membrane, with the prosthetic ring

b. Making the Matrix

The array was fabricated on a machine called "Vertical Machining Center". It is nothing more than a machine tool with computer numerical control. Utilizing cutting tool, and stainless steel plant directly. Figures: 5,6,7

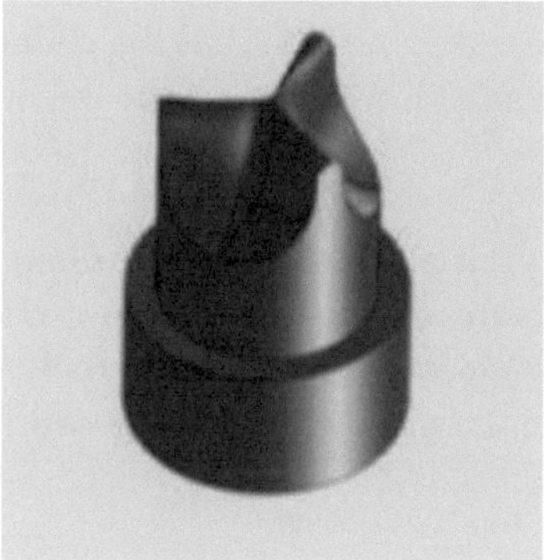

Figure 5. Matrix made of stainless steel

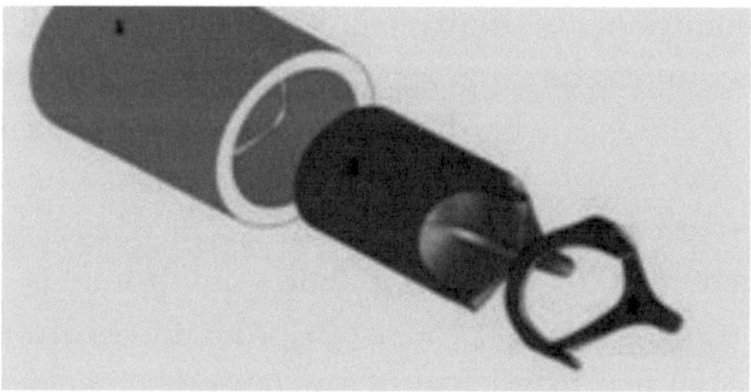

Figure 6. Coupling ring in the matrix and stainless steel support

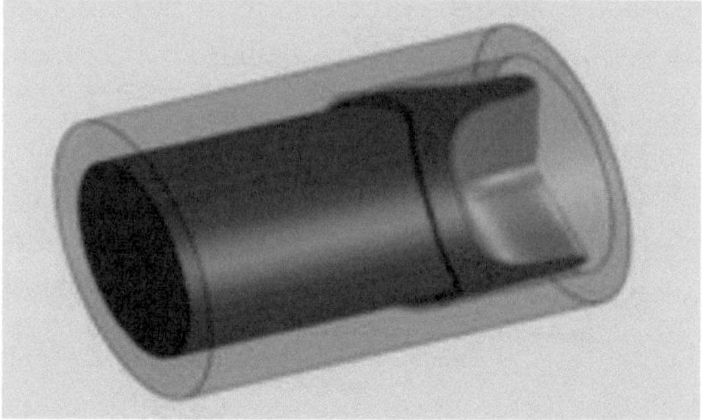

Figure 7. Coupling of the matrix to the ring and support for the filling with *segmented polyurethane (SPU)*

c. Manufacturing segmented polyurethane prostheses

Among the polymeric materials used in clinical practice, *polyurethanes* have paved their place in the market and are the best choice for application in the field of medical implants. Present biostability, biocompatibility, high lubricity, strength, abrasion resistance and fatigue is also easy to use, presenting flexibility and resistance to thromboembolism. These are some of the reasons why *polyurethanes* are used for a variety of medical devices. To develop a prosthetic heart it will be necessary to use a polymer that has the characteristics described above, it is necessary hemodynamic and biophysical testing to rate the quality of the material.

- Polyurethanes

Thermoplastic *polyurethanes* exhibit a wide range of technological applications due to the versatility of the chemical structure and properties that can be achieved from various commercially available *diisocyanates* and *alkanediols*. Additionally, the physical properties achievable in these materials can be enlarged by the relative concentrations of the raw materials capable of producing polymers.

The *polyurethanes* exhibit microphase separated structure comprising soft segments and hard segments. The flexible segments are formed usually from oligomers with long segments such as *methylene, oxy-alkylene,* or other *aliphatic* sequence, while the hard segment is formed by *urethanic* segments resulting from the reaction of short chain *alkanediols* and *diisocyanates*. The highly polar nature of the urethane linkages is responsible for the thermodynamics of phase separation micro-heterogeneous, which together with the possibility of formation of crystalline phase in the hard and soft phases, make complex relations between these various domains and the physical and mechanical behavior observed. Additionally, it is noted that the formation of these domains in *polyurethanes* is also a function of its processing, since, in general, the thermodynamic equilibrium is not achieved in these materials during their transformation process. In order to ensure consistent performance of the product it is essential that its microstructure does not change significantly with time. Thus, for applications with high demands is the use of appropriate heat treatment, annealing, and the environmental application similar to the use of the product, where in contact with blood, subjected to cyclic strain. It is noteworthy that the use of dynamic mechanical thermal analysis allows detailed tracking of transformations undergone by the product according to the process of thermal annealing and contact with fluid.

d. Manufacturing prostheses by injection of PCU matrix

In this design, it is intended to prepare *polyurethane* membranes from different sources using the techniques of hot pressing and evaporation of the solution. Prepare membranes with different thicknesses in the range of 50 to 200 *um*. These membranes are subjected to thermal annealing treatments in idealized fluids simulating blood.

The membranes obtained under different conditions are identified, using the techniques of X-ray diffractometry, differential scanning calorimetry and dynamic mechanical thermal analysis, among others. Additionally, ultrasound technique allows the analysis for the presence of defects in 100% of the membranes to be employed in the construction of prosthetic heart *polyurethane.* Figure 8.

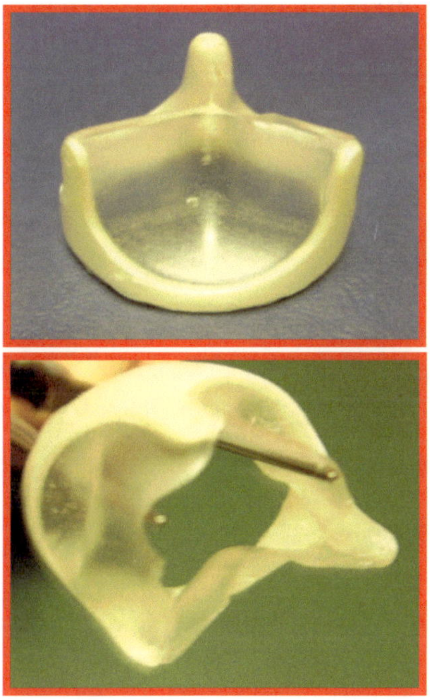

Figure 8. Prototype of *Segmented Polyurethane(SPU)* prosthesis.

3. Discussion

3.1. Durability of *polyurethane* prosthesis tested *"in vitro"*

The *SPU* prostheses have shown a useful life of over 130 million cycles in real time and 420 million cycles at accelerated conditions without failure of the *SPU* [13]. *In vivo* conditions, the longest period after implantation was 399 days, performing euthanasia due to the excessive growth of the animal. [13] In summary, these data demonstrate the good hemodynamic performance behavior of the implanted SPU prosthesis right side of the heart, in particular lack of a significant pressure gradient after 1 year of implantation. This study confirms the good biocompatibility of *SPU* (low thrombogenicity in animals without anticoagulant therapy) and short-term durability of such compounds without the use of anti-calcification in a model of accelerated mineralization.

Author details

Miguel A. Maluf[1], Hector A. Barone[2] and Fabricio Sena[3]

1 Cardiovascular Division, Universidade Federal de São Paulo, Brazil

2 Industrias Barone, Campinas, São Paulo, Brazil

3 Empresa Rone, São Paulo, Brazil

References

[1] Danielson GK, Anderson BJ, Schleck CD, Ilstrup DM. Late results of pulmonary ventricle to pulmonary artery conduits. *Semin Thorac Cardiovasc Surg 1995;17:162-7.*

[2] Kirklin JW, Blackstone EH, Maehara T, Pacifico AD, Pollock S, Stewart RW. Intermediate-term fate of cryopreserved allograft and xenograft valved conduits. *Ann Thorac Surg 1987;44:598-606.*

[3] Hawkins JA, Bailey WW, Dillon T, Schwartz DC. Midterm results with cryopreserved allograft valved conduits from the right ventricle to the pulmonary arteries. *J Thorac Cardiovasc Surg 1992;104:910-6.*

[4] Cleveland DC, Williams W, Razzouk AJ, et al. Failure of cryopreserved homograft valved conduits in the pulmonary circulation. *Circulation 1992;86(suppl):II150-3.*

[5] Boyce SW, Turley K, Yee ES, Verrier ED, Ebert PA. The fate of the 12 mm porcine valved conduit from the right ventricle to the pulmonary artery: a ten-year experience. *J Thorac Cardiovasc Surg 1988;95:201-7.*

[6] Sano S, Karl TR, Mee RB. Extracardiac valved conduits in the pulmonary circuit. *Ann Thorac Surg 1991;52:285-90.*

[7] McGoon DC, Danielson GK, Puga FJ, Ritter DG, Mair DD, Ilstrup DM. Late results after extracardiac conduit repair for congenital cardiac defects. *Am J Cardiol 1982;49:1741-9.*

[8] Maluf MA, Braile DM, Silva C, Catani R, Carvalho AC, Buffolo E: Reconstruction of the pulmonary valve and right ventricular outflow tract with bicuspid prosthesis in tetralogy of Fallot. *Ann Thorac Surg 2000;70:1911-1917*

[9] Miguel Maluf; Antonio Carvalho; Werther Carvalho Use of Right Ventricular Remodeling Surgery with a Porcine Pulmonary Prosthesis for Congenital Heart Disease. *The Heart Surgery Forum 2011; 14 (1); E40-E50*

[10] Miguel Maluf - Late outcome of right ventricular outflow tract repair using bicuspid pulmonary prosthesis in tetralogy of Fallot surgery repair: case report. *Rev Bras Cir Cardiovasc 2009;24(4): 574-577.*

[11] Champsaur G, Ninet J, Vigneron M, Neidecker J, Boissonat P. Use of the ABIOMED BVS System 5000 as a bridge to cardiac transplantation. *J Thorac Cardiovasc Surg 1990;100:122-8*

[12] Lederman DM. Technical considerations in the development of clinical systems for temporary and permanent cardiac support. In: Unger F, editor. *Assisted circulation. Berlin: Springer Verlag; 1984. p. 115-27.*

[13] Yu LS, Finnegan M, Vaughan S, et al. A compact and noise free electrohydraulic total artificial heart. *ASAIO J 1993;39:M386-91*

[14] Sabine H. Daebritz, Jörg S. Sachweh, Benita Hermanns, Bernd Fausten, Andreas Franke, Jan Groetzner, Bernd Klosterhalfen, Bruno J. Messmer. Introduction of a Flexible Polymeric Heart Valve Prosthesis With Special Design for Mitral Position. *Circulation.* 2003; 108: II-134-II-139

Chapter 2

Adult Cardiopulmonary Bypass in the Twenty-First Century — Science, Art or Empiricism?

Paulo Roberto Barbosa Evora and
Alfredo José Rodrigues

Additional information is available at the end of the chapter

http://dx.doi.org/10.5772/57108

1. Introduction

Among all surgery modalities known today, the heart surgery was one of the few that only in the last century has become bravely discovered by surgeons, and the always gone toward safe ways due to the tenacity and commitment of several scientists. The cardiopulmonary bypass (CPB) was the responsible for the achievement of this status because due to this procedure, the heart surgeries have become safer and some more complex defects could be approached.

This chapter aims to highlight some little discussed aspects of the CPB, taking into account physiology and physiopathology aspects and some new perfusion technologies.

The first of these aspects concerns to the fact that the surgeons no longer worried about the CPB, since the perfusionists began to make a quality support, besides the technical performance of the procedure. Therefore, the surgeons must maintain and update their knowledge about CPB due to the simple fact of maintaining its educational leadership over their team. On the other hand, it seems that there is certain complacency in relation to the CPB since, in recent times, the quality of the CPB apparatus ensures a strong safety for heart operations.

The second aspect concerns an intriguing detail. The CPB techniques are clearly distinct into protocols for children and protocols for adults. Among adults would not be appealing the preparation of protocols individually? For example, the elderly and diabetics, due to their individual characteristics, would not deserve more appropriate protocols?

The third motivational aspect of this review may be the questioning of so harmful systemic inflammatory reaction caused by exposure of blood to the non endothelized surface of the CPB circuits. Due the fact that the inflammatory response is present in patients undergone off-pump surgery, the focus has changed to the concept that, more than the contact with the CPB circuit, the contact of the blood with the operatory wound may be the most responsible by the inflammation phenomenon in CPB. This even induced to the consideration of the contact of the blood with serous membranes (pleura and pericardium), which have, as well known, fibrinolytic activity as a cause of increased bleeding. Thus, the maintenance of the pleural integrity in the dissection of the internal thoracic arteries has become an attractive detail of surgical technique.

Finally, what is the motivation for the review title? Regarding the CPB in its current patterns, would it be a consequence of empiricism or science? We are convinced that both empiricism and science are extremely strong. Thus, the greatest motivation of this review was to provide knowledge in order that the teams involved in cardiac surgeries may standardize their knowledge about CPB and pursuit the enhancement of the scientific aspects that guide the procedure.

2. Microcirculation

The cardiovascular system is a complex set of vessels, within which the blood circulates through the body, pumped by the heart. In this way, the veins are responsible for the flow in centripetal way, whereas the arteries are responsible for the flow in centrifugal way. Interposed between the distal arterial and venous territories are the constituents of the microcirculation, composed of arterioles, capillaries and venules. It deals with the exchanges between the blood and tissues under the regulatory mechanisms of peripheral blood flow. The flow regulation in the capillary bed occurs by means of the arteriovenous communications - which can deflect the blood from the capillaries - and by means of the pre- and postcapillaries sphincters, which actions control the blood volume and the pressure in the capillary bed. The flow control in the microcirculation complies to metabolic changes as for both hormonal or neural stimuli [1]. We can emphasize that, during the CPB, the circulation physiology is totally modified by the introduction of a non pulsatile flow of the arterial side that differs from a high venous pressure on the venous side of the circulation (Figure 1). This situation induces to adaptation mechanisms and those main are represented in Figure 2.

2.1. Adaptation mechanisms

Throughout all their extension, the components of the cardiovascular system are coated by three basic tissue layers, suffering variations on the thickness in the different types of vessels that constitute the system. These layers are: a) intimal layer, more internal, consisting of endothelium, which the primary function is to avoid contact of blood with endothelial thrombogenic substances b) thickness of the media layer, consisting (in more or less intensity) of elastic and muscle tissue and; c) Adventitia or external layer, primarily composed of conjunctive tissue [1.2].

In the pressure gradient found along the circulation, the pressure has a greater value in the left ventricle reaching (during the systole), the mean value of 120 mmHg, decreasing then in

http://dx.doi.org/10.5772/57108

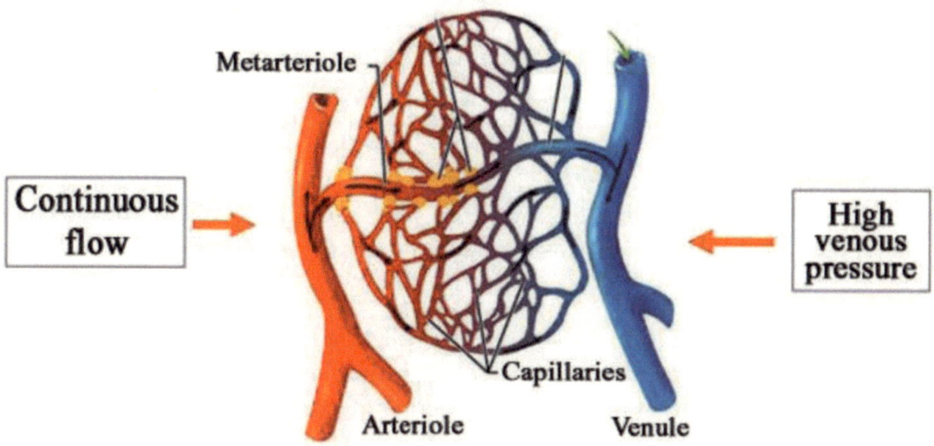

Figure 1. Microcirculation in cardiopulmonary bypass (CPB)

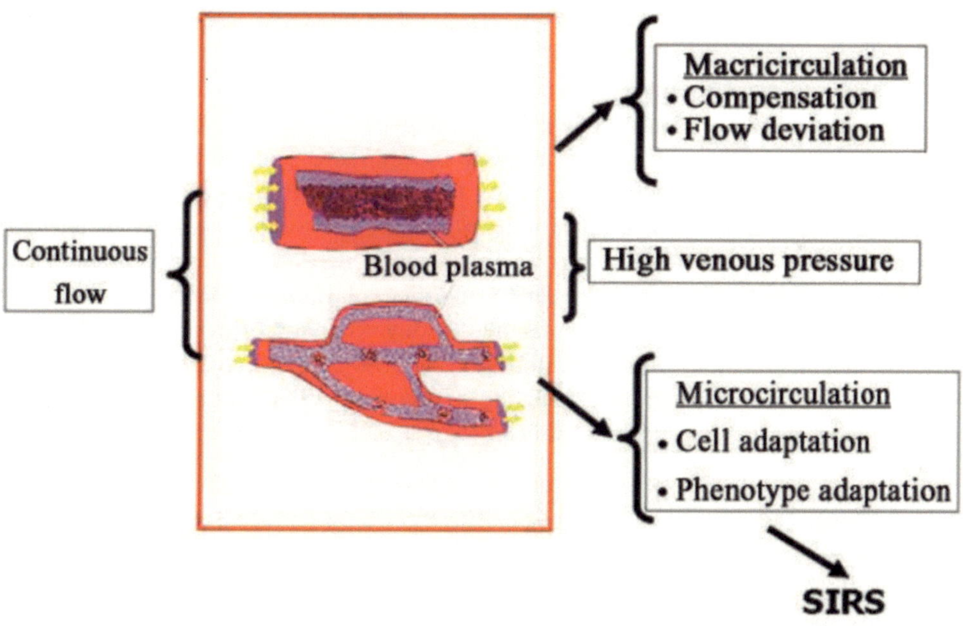

Figure 2. Microcirculation in cardiopulmonary bypass (CPB)

the diastole and reaching around 0 mmHg. At the aortic root, the systolic pressure has the same value found in the heart. However, the diastolic pressure decreases to around 80 mmHg. It may be explained by the storage of energy imposed by the blood on the arterial wall during the systole and released during the diastole, ensuring the flow throughout all cardiac cycle. In the distal arteries, both values of systolic or diastolic pressure decrease in relation to the origin of the aorta, as well as the pressure and pulse (that is the difference between the systolic and diastolic pressure).

The pulse pressure reaches zero value from the capillary territory, and the difference between the pressure of the arteriolar extremity (about 40 mmHg) and the venous extremity (about 20 mmHg) creates a decreasing pressure gradient along the capillary. In the return to the heart along the venous system, the blood pressure gradually decreases until reaching a value around zero in the right atrium [2].

The microcirculation morphology is not uniform in all organs of the body, thus, in the central nervous system, in the lungs, skin and the skeletal muscle the capillary endothelium is of continuous type. The intestinal mucous, the exocrine glands, the renal glomerulus and the choroid plexus are composed of fenestrated-type endothelium. Finally in the liver, spleen and bone marrow, the endothelium is of discontinuous type [2]. The microcirculation flow is non pulsatile as in the arteries, because the pulse pressure in the territory is null. Moreover, the flow in capillaries is intermittent because the contraction in the pre-capillaries sphincters may block the passage of blood during rest, allowing that the capillaries may oscillate opening and closing.

The use of cardiopulmonary bypass (that in the majority of cases occurs with non pulsatile flow) is considered harmful to the microcirculation, thus providing a "shunting" effect. Moreover, the technique is responsible for other changes in circulation, such as a replacement of reflex and chemoreceptors controls; increase of venous pressure; decreasing of colloid osmotic pressure and manipulated temperature. The replacement of the physiological controls induces the capillary flow not be intermittent and to be continuous instead, which increases the pressure on the venous side forcing - in the microcirculation - the performance of compensation mechanisms for flow deviation. In the microcirculation, the continuous flow induces to phenotypic cell adaptation that results in the development of systemic inflammatory response syndrome (SIRS) [2]. Once initiated this response occurs activation of inflammatory cells and triggering the coagulation cascade It also occurs the release of cell signaling protein, generation of vasoactive and, cytotoxic substances associated to the production of a diversity of microembolus.

Another way of microcirculation lesion related to the use of CPB is the formation of microbubbles that circulate in the blood flow and lodge in the capillaries causing obstruction, promoting ischemia, inflammation, complement activation, platelet aggregation and formation of blood clots [3].

In last decades, occurred considerable advances in CPB equipment in order to avoid the development of SIRS. This achievement has had some success, but we cannot affirm the same regarding to microcirculation lesion. The damage caused in the microcirculation can be evidenced by the detection of products of several organs degradation that is, undoubtedly, an important function to help the perfusionists to improve their techniques. One of the markers that may meet this function may be the "mitogen-activated protein kinases" (MAPK) that have been involved in the vasomotor function since the microcirculation regulation includes the miogenic tone [4].

3. CPB monitoring

Up to now, there is no method for monitoring of the regional perfusion during the CPB, which leads to the question about which markers could be used to determine the adequacy of arterial flow during the CPB. A discussion about possible parameters that may meet this purpose is here presented as follows. This discussion was presented by one of the authors (PRBE), in 2007, in the 34th Congress of the Brazilian Society of Cardiovascular Surgery [2].

3.1. Oxygen partial pressure of venous blood (PvO2) and venous saturation of venous blood (SvO2)

The SvO2 presents some problems, among them, the fact that if the distant capillaries are not equally perfused, tissues may not receive appropriate flows resulting in an increase of the PVO2 or SVO2, mimicking a vascular shunt. Thus, the PVO2 or SVO2, despite the fact that they are markers easy to be measured, they may not be related to the appropriate tissue perfusion, not necessarily suggesting that the cell oxygenation is satisfactory [5].

3.2. Lactate

Among the problems presented by the lactate, we may mention that the release of this substance in the blood demands blood flow; thus, high levels may be typically identified later in the postoperative [5]. For the measurement of intraoperative lactate, the lactate/pyruvate relationship may be a better method, but requires additional analytical instrumentation. The systemic microvascular control may be disordered in the non pulsatile CPB. This disorder causes "shunting" and increases lactate despite an apparent oxygen supply. Extreme hemodilution, hypothermia, low flow of CPB and excessive neuronal activation have been related to lactic acidosis during CPB.

3.3. Partial pressure gradients of carbon dioxide between the venous and arterial blood samples ("PCO2)

The PCO2 gradient between the arterial and venous blood samples (Ä PCO2) is a valuable parameter for determining the adequacy of the CPB for a certain metabolic condition and may help to detect alterations in oxygen demand (metabolic alterations that accompany the temperature changes, CPB flows and drugs administration). Amongst the SvO2, which is valuable patient's metabolic index during CPB, the Ä PCO2 can help to fulfill the role in the adequacy of the tissue perfusion during surgery. This gradient, perhaps one of the best parameters of tissue perfusion is rarely used by perfusionists perhaps due to its lack of knowledge.

3.4. Arterial pressure

An arterial pressure is extremely powerful in determining the adequacy of CPB. However, it is difficult to establish what pressure level may indicate a best perfusion for each patient and their physiopathological particularities.

4. Technologies

The introduction of CPB apparatus has solved obstacles that did not allow access to the inner cavity of the heart; however, this fact revealed a myriad of complications from the response of the organism to the aggressions imposed by the apparatus. Thus, throughout the years after the introduction of the CPB, a paradoxical and new situation of a number of complications related to the use of CPB were observed. Among these problems, the main are: a) the severe inflammatory response that the patients develop when their blood are exposed to nonendothelial surface of the apparatus, b) the excessive hemodilution or the need of use of homologous blood to fill the circuit, and c) the microcirculation lesion caused by the flow imposed by the apparatus pumps.

Some technologies have been developed, modernly, aiming at the resolution of these problems. Herein, we will approach some of these major advances.

4.1. Retrograde autologous priming

Since the creation of CPB, the cardiac surgeries present high risk for blood transfusion, due to possible bleeding inherent to the surgery. The CPB circuit should be filled adding crystalloid solutions to remove the air system resulting many times in severe hemodilution. Initially, homologous blood was used for this purpose, but the risk of disease transmission and the lack of donors contributed to search for alternative materials. The introduction of crystalloid substances to fill the circuit (the called "pattern technique") solved that question, but the frequent severe hemodilution induces to the need of new transfusions. Moreover, the hemodilution presents undesirable effects such as decreasing of the blood osmotic pressure and its inability to carry oxygen causing acidosis, hypoxia, edema and clotting alterations [6]. Studies evaluating the hemodilution effects showed an association with high rates of mortality and other adverse conditions, which occur mostly when the hematocrit levels are lesser than 20%. The low hematocrits during the CPB are associated to an increase of hospital mortality risks, need of use of an intra-aortic balloon in per or postoperative and the need to return to the perfusion after the end of CPB. In addition to these results, ethical and religious pressures against blood transfusions, the scarcity of material and the risk of disease transmission, induce to search alternatives to fill the system.

The resolution for these problems was attempted by the introduction of a new technique, the Retrograde Autologous Priming (RAP), described initially by Panico and Neptune [7] in 1959, and adapted later by several authors [5,8,9]. The basic idea consists of filling the CPB circuit with the patient's own blood. To this end, the circuit is initially filled with crystalloid solution and then, allowing that the blood retrogradely flows from the aorta of the patient to the arterial line, moving part of the acellular prime that was in the arterial line to the bag collector. After that, the forceps of the venous line are opened allowing the venous blood drainage of the patient. At the same time, the arterial pump is slowly moved in order to maintain a constant liquid level in the venous reservoir. Then, the blood moves the remaining solution of the circuit to the bag and the CPB may be initiated. If there is a need of liquid addition during the perfusion, the prime stored in the collector bags can be introduced in the circuit by means of the recirculation line. The technique of RAP has proved to be a safe, low cost and highly effective in reducing the hemodilution associated to the heart surgery. This provides a blood viscosity closer to the physiological blood, does not change the values of plasmatic proteins, contributing to a better balance in osmotic pressure and reduction of edema. Moreover, the technique does not compromise the function of the clotting factors and the vessel-regulator hormones. As previously mentioned, the technique reduces the need of blood transfusions and allows the control of the hematocrit to reach the intended levels by manipulating the amount of crystalloid released by the backup bags.

The use of the technique allows less hemodynamic instability and rapid perfusion initiation. The potential risks of the use of RAP technique are related to the reduction of hemodilution, because the patients who are under hypothermia may present increase in the blood viscosity about 10% to 30%. This can be solved by a moderate hemodilution during the procedure, avoiding microcirculation impairment.

4.2. Pulsatile flow

The blood arterial flow in the organism is a pulsatile type, or that is, with changes in pressure during systolic and diastolic phases; however, since its invention, the CPB determines a non pulsatile flow, or that is, the pressure does not undergo significant variations over the perfusion. This difference raised the suspicion that pulsatile blood flow may provide a most appropriate and less harmful perfusion inducing a series of comparative studies between the two systems. Promising results showing hemodynamic and metabolic improvement -compared to the conventional method - point to the pulsatile flow as an important tool to reduce complications associated with the use of CPB [10-12].

It was suggested that the most benefic effect of the use of pulsatile flow may be in the territory of the microcirculation, where the energy of the pulsatile flow eases the interstitial diffusion by the oscillation of cell membranes and promotes the arterioles patency (which remain collapsed during the non pulsatile flow). In addition to this is the fact that the continued opening of arterioles reduces the stress produced by the decreased release of endothelial vasodilators.

Although the literature presents conflicting data, many researchers have shown that the pulsatile flow improves cerebral blood flow as well as avoiding the drop of renal function and tubular changes found during the use of non pulsatile flow. Moreover, it was demonstrated that the use of the technique increases the urine output and reduces proteinuria. It seems logical that the pulsatile flow is beneficial or even needful to maintain the body's physiological state. Therefore, in order to the extracorporeal support system may mimic the characteristics of pressure and flow as close as possible of the physiological characteristics, it need to seek the exact wave type needed to reach a satisfactory pulsatile flow by the artificial pumps. This is a controversial aspect, since there are defenders that only the presence of any pulse already shows benefic effects.

4.3. Minicircuits

The severe inflammatory response associated with the materials used in CPB apparatus has raised the idea that the reduction of the size of circuits may reduce the degree of this response and minimize the harmful effects of the CPB; moreover, minor apparatus may reduce the prime quantity needed and may minimize the hemodilution and the need for homologous transfusions.

The concept of mini-CPB combines the known clinical advantages of the impregnated circuits, reduction of the prime volume and reuse of the aspirated blood from the surgical field. These circuits are composed of a centrifugal pump, a membrane oxygenator, a heat exchanger, a "cell saver" system for blood collection from the surgical field and an arterial filter, due to the higher risk of air entering that these systems have [13].

Initially created to be used in CABG; throughout time and with increasing experience of the teams, the mini-CPB has been showing increasingly useful, expanding the number of indications for more complex procedures and replacing the conventional systems. A comparative study between patients undergone conventional system and mini-CPB revealed some number of microbubbles in the conventional system increasing the chances of these patients to develop cognitive deficits [14]. Another study of the same nature revealed that the use of mini-CPB's reduces hemodilution and thus the need for homologous transfusions associated to the procedure. These observations in the study were associated with postoperative bleeding reductions.

Despite the small number, the studies related to the new system have been showing superiority in the benefits of minicircuits in relation to conventional systems up to now. Future studies should be made to expand the indications on its use in a larger number of procedures.

4.4. Impregnated circuits

The interaction between the blood and nonendothelial surfaces of the CPB circuit is responsible for the development of severe inflammatory response based on the activation of complement and the kallikrein system. In addition to that, the release of cytokines contributes to severe complications in the peri and postoperative and increases the surgical morbidity and mortality. These problems can be solved by means of materials that allow the biocompatibility to the system, or that is, materials that avoid the deleterious effects of nonendothelial materials of the apparatus in contact with the patient's blood. It was proven that the heparin, commonly used due to its antithrombotic properties, is capable of providing properties of biocompatibility, inhibiting by the contact the activation of complement and adsorbing lipoproteins to create a surface that mimics the cell membranes.

The use of heparin in the coating of the CPB apparatus has proved to be capable to reduce blood loss, as well as the need for blood transfusions or derivatives. Moreover, the achieved reduction of inflammatory response has benefic effects on the patient's clinical evolution. Mangoush et al. [15] also showed that the substance reduced the ventilation time in 78 minutes, as well as the hospitalization time in 0.5 days. Because of these reductions, the use of the mentioned substance also allows overriding economy in terms of financial costs.

Phosphorylcholine is a coating that allows system biocompatibility. This phospholipid is frequently associated to a copolymer (methacryloyl- phosphorylcholine/lauryl-methacrylate (MPC:LM). Its characteristics allow coating of other polymers, showing stability and little waste by leaching. It has proved that the coating resists to the fibrinogen adsorption, connection and activation of platelets [16, 17]. The effects on the clinical status of the patient still need further studies, but in the few performed studies were found the reduction of immediate postoperative bleeding, preservation of platelets and a positive effect on the generation of complement.

A third group of products is also commercially available and involves the concept of "microdomains" to minimize the interactions between the surface, the cells and the proteins. The new technology uses copolymers, from which hydrophobic and hydrophilic "microdomains" are interchanged on the surface of contact with blood. The control of the distances among these "microdomains" allows them to compete among themselves ("microdomain" inhibiting effect of another), which limits the adsorption of protein [18].

The cell membranes of circulating leukocytes and platelets is also under the same competitive interaction between the surface and the membrane constituents minimizing the cellular connection. A few clinical studies have shown inhibition of the generation of thrombin and fibrinolysis during the use of these coatings. Moreover, there is protection of platelets with reduction of their activation.

Some other materials are commercially available, but almost all of them still requiring more studies to confirm their benefits. Future advances in materials engineering focusing the search of products with high biocompatibility will allow better results in reducing complications by the use of CPB.

5. Cardiopulmonary bypass in elderly

In recent years, world population is going through an "aging process". This increase of the elderly population additionally brings increase of the prevalence of diseases inherent to this age-group, among them the cardiovascular diseases. As a result, the heart surgery in elderly is increasing, and some procedures, such as CABG, correction of valve lesions (specially the aortic valve), and repair of aneurysms and dissections of the aorta are becoming common.

The peculiarities of this population bring as a challenge to patients selection the adoption of peri- and postoperative cares, and the choice of surgical techniques that reduce the morbidity and mortality in those patients. As elderly patients may undergone to high-risk surgical procedures it is necessary to understand the physiological alterations, in order to prevent no complications as early as possible. In addition, it is crucial to consider the expectation and quality of life that intervention will bring to the patient [18, 19].

Some physiological aspects of aging involve in well known particularities such as cardiovascular, lung and kidney physiologies, which are extremely valuable for the CPB planning. These particularities of the elderly physiology justify one of the initial propositions of this study (special protocols for elderly), motivating also the pursuit for excellence in pre- and perioperative care of these patients. Preexisting diseases have a greater impact on morbidity and mortality than this age for itself. Meanwhile, although the age alone does not constitute a risk factor for heart surgery, it may not be an extreme the individualization of CPB protocols for elderly [18, 19].

The preparation of the CPB does not differ significantly from the perfusion for adults in general, however, taking into account that the elderly is characterized by reduced organic reserves, it needs higher stability during perfusion. The peculiarities of the elderly include higher systolic pressure due to greater rigidity of the arteries, reduction of the blood flow brain and lower oxygen consumption by the tissues. Also, due to higher incidence of neurological complications by microembolia, it is recommended the use of the filter in the arterial line. Other recommendations include maintaining blood pressure at higher levels than the average 70-80 mmHg at all stages of the infusion; the hematocrit between 25 and 30% and an oncotic normal pressure, which is obtained by adding synthetic colloids, plasma or albumin, avoiding cerebral and pulmonary edema. Concerning to the temperature, is preferable the normothermia or rapid hypothermia [20].

6. Cardiopulmonary bypass in the diabetic patient

Diabetic patients undergoing on-pump heart surgery present increased rate of severe complications. The oxidative stress is about two times high in diabetics. Furthermore, some studies have reported that the inflammatory response is different when the two groups are compared. Despite not yet entirely known, the metabolism of nitric oxide (NO) was involved as participating of these alterations. The different possible mechanisms already outline therapeutic possibilities to reduce the deleterious effects of the CPB in these patients.

The suspicion that the NO may be involved in the physiopathology related to the use of CPB motivated many studies, many of them comparing different parameters between diabetics and nondiabetic patients. Matata and Galiñanes performed a study in which they measured the stable metabolites levels of NO (NOx) in urine and blood. These metabolites are the main way of NO degradation and due the fact that they do not suffer immediate degradation, their measurement is a reliable indication of the production of NO. The results showed that NOx levels are already high in basal conditions, in the diabetic group, explaining the greater susceptibility to oxidative stress. Moreover, the levels of these metabolites suffer significant additional increase during heart surgery that was not observed in the nondiabetic group [21, 22].

It is known that the reaction between NO and the superoxide anions induces to the formation of powerful oxidizing peroxynitrite (ONOO-), which can exacerbate the oxidative stress in diabetics. Those peroxynitrites are the main generators of hydroxyl radicals that can cause serious lesions and cell death. Moreover, the free radicals generated during the CPB induce to peroxidation of lipids and proteins that change the enzyme activity. Based on the fact that the pretreatment with antioxidants before the CPB reduces oxidative attack, interventions with antioxidants may represent possible therapeutic aim.

It is suspected that the cause of increase of NO is the increased expression of inducible NO synthase (iNOS) in these patients [21]. The suspicions of implication of the NO in the physiopathology of the adverse events observed after CPB has induced studies about NO donors. Moreover, these substances are usually used to hemodynamic control during and after CPB, and the effects of exogenous NO on oxidation and inflammatory response concerning the clinical status of patients were unknown.

These studies showed that exogenous NO significantly reduced the oxidative stress in diabetic patients and differently affected inflammatory response [22]. In these two groups of patients, the use of NO donors decreased the formation of nitrotyrosine protein, but only in diabetics there was a significant reduction in formation of lipid hydroperoxides and protein carbonylation. These observations may be explained by the reduction of formation of endogenous NO by means of exogenous NO. Thus, the results showed that exogenous NO seems to present a powerful antioxidant activity in humans, which may allow the extension of its use to the usual hemodynamic control.

Alteration in NOx levels also were compared in response to the administration of nitroglycerin (TNG), revealing that this substance, in accordance with the findings described above, is also able to reduce significantly urinary and plasmatic levels of NOx in diabetics. One hypothesis about the way the TNG exerts this effect on NO metabolism may be by the negative regulation on the activity of constitutive NOS. Another possibility may be that the TNG reduces the capture of L-arginine (precursor of NO) by cells, emphasizing that the two mechanisms are not mutually exclusive and may occur together, inducing the reduction of the NOx levels in diabetics [22].

Study about the use of TNG on the inflammatory response [21] showed that this drug increased the IL-8 levels, and plasma elastase in diabetics, whilst in nondiabetic group there increased complements activation. These findings show that the inflammatory response in diabetic patients is different from the response in nondiabetics and, moreover, the answer to the TNG is also different between the two groups.

There are also reports of minor hospital stay (marginally not significant) in diabetic patients who received TNG, although it increases the release of some components of the inflammatory response of CPB in both groups of patients. Thus, despite the benefits, the increase of the inflammatory response observed by NO donor drugs regarding to their use - requires care, especially in patients under proinflammatory conditions.

Other studies have shown a reduction in the complement activation to the use of another NO donor (sodium nitroprusside) [23]. This may indicate that the donor type and the time of use, as well as, the dose of administration may be beneficial in determining the effect of these agents in the inflammatory cascade. Thus, as the oxidative stress is increased in diabetic patients, its reduction, by NO donors, may be a possible therapy.

6.1. Vasoplegia in diabetics

Another adverse effect of the use of CPB is the vasoplegic syndrome, which is characterized by the appearance of severe hypotension, reduction in systemic vascular resistance and arteriolar reactivity, increase of need for volume replacement and vasopressor therapy, and appropriate or high cardiac output. Nitric oxide mediators were discovered as participants of this syndrome, allowing also some therapies. Few studies characterize this syndrome in diabetics and, as previously discussed, diabetics present an altered NO metabolism; moreover, some differences in control of perfusion regulation between the two groups of patients are known [24].

The alterations presented in healthy patients along surgery induced to an increase in the pCO2 concentrations, acetylcholine, ADP, that with hypoxia stimulate the NOS to produce NO, which function is to regulate the flow by means of vasodilation. In diabetics, the changes that occur in this flow regulation mechanism are characterized by insufficient production of NO, despite the presence of appropriate stimuli on the NOS. This effect sums to the thickening of the basal membrane and may block the passage of the little remainder NO that was produced, avoiding that it may reach the vascular smooth muscle and exerts its vasodilator effect [25].

7. Inflammatory reaction and vasoplegic syndrome associated to cardiopulmonary bypass

The physiopathology of post-CPB vasoplegia is multifactorial, with no final consensus on its real mechanism. The emphasis will be on systemic inflammatory reaction with possible "trigger" from the contact of blood with nonendothelial surfaces of CPB and the possible mechanism related to the vasopressin deficiency.

7.1. Systemic inflammatory reaction

The modern era of heart surgery had its beginning when the CPB technique was introduced in the beginnings of 50' decade. The CPB is essential for the majority of cardiac surgeries, but an undesirable inflammatory reaction occurs as a result of its use. To understand the vasoplegic syndrome physiopathology there are many hypotheses including a) viral and bacterial infections b) immunological reactions related to anti myocardial antibodies c) anaphylactoid reactions associated to anesthetics, protamine, heparin and the CPB circuit itself [26].

Many factors during the CPB, dependent (exposure of blood to surfaces and not physiological conditions) or independent of the CPB material (surgical trauma, ischemia-reperfusion of the organs, changes in body temperature and release of endotoxins), have been reported as inducers of a complex inflammatory response. These factors include the activation of the complement system, release of cytokines, leukocyte activation and the expression of adhesion molecules, in addition to the production of various substances, such as oxygen free radicals, arachidonic acid metabolites, platelet-activating factor (PAF), NO and endothelins. Such inflammatory cascade may contribute to the development of postoperative complications, including respiratory failure, renal dysfunction, hemorrhagic disorders, neurological dysfunction, changes in liver function, and finally failure of multiple organs. More recently, it was observed that this antiinflammatory response may initiate during and after CPB. This complex chain of events has strong similarities with sepsis.

For the CPB circuit, it can be emphasized that its incidence is higher with the use of bubble oxygenators in relation to the membrane oxygenators. Its real physiopathology remains unclear and may be described a logical sequence of events: proinflammatory and/or inflammatory stimuli with activation of the complement system; release of various cytokines (interleukins, tumor necrosis factor, platelet activating factor, etc.); activation of the inducible nitric oxide synthase (iNOS); production of NO; activation of guanylate cyclase with an increase of cyclic GMP which leads to the refractory vasoplegia even to the use of high doses of adrenergic amines. There is also a tendency for diffuse bleeding by the NO antiplatelet activities of NO [26]. The schematic representation of this inflammatory response can be observed in Figure 3. Regarding the NO participation, it is curious to observe that a clinical study measuring nitrates in urine and blood of patients undergone on-pump heart surgery, has not shown a correlation between endogenous NO and low systemic vascular resistance [27].

In relation to the individually involved mechanisms, some data worth highlighting:

1. The clinical relevance of the complement activation itself is still uncertain. Several studies have linked the postoperative morbidity to the complement activation;

2. The prevention of neutrophils adhesion may bring practical benefits, but these benefits may be associated to a greater risk of infection;

3. The leukocytes activation may release large amounts of oxygen free radicals, including the superoxide anion, hydrogen peroxide, hydroxyl radical and the oxygen itself. These radicals act on lipidic membranes by increasing the permeability which can involve the cardiac and pulmonary functions;

4. The metabolism products of arachidonic acid (prostaglandins, leukotrienes and thromboxane A2) may be counterbalanced by the concomitant production of vasodilators prostaglandins such as the prostacyclin (PGI2). The leukotrienes may be responsible for the increase of capillary permeability;

5. Endotoxin levels may increase during and after CPB. The sources of endotoxins are highly diverse. However, the most significant source is related to the intestines. The splanchnic vasoconstriction during the CPB may induce to ischemia and increase of the permeability of intestinal loops with the release of endotoxins into the blood flow. The endotoxins levels are related to the initial vasoconstriction, time of aortic clamping and hypo-oncotic state during the CPB;

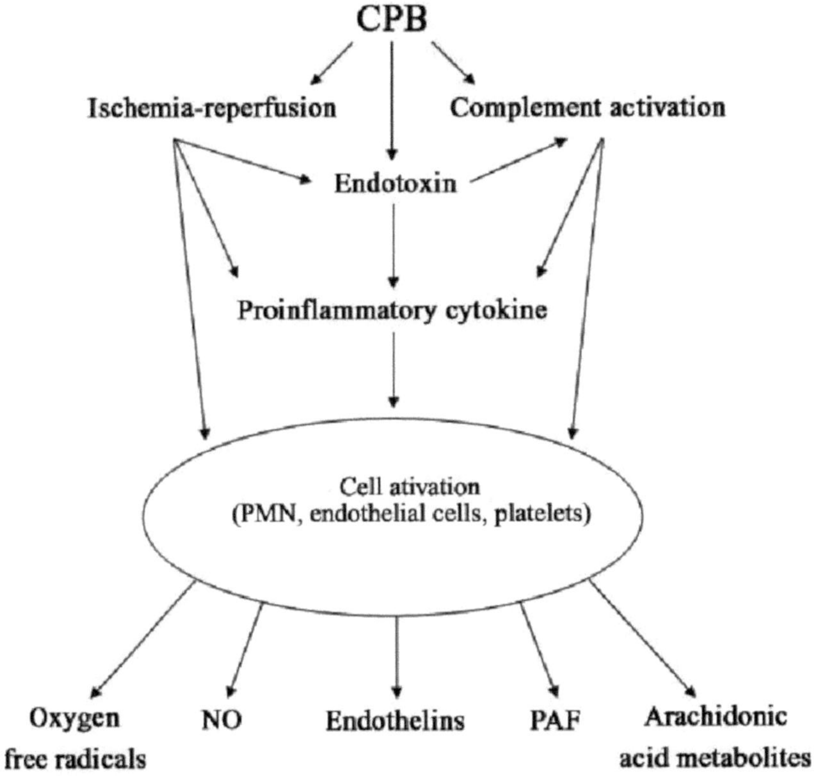

Figure 3. Outline of the inflammatory response generated by cardiopulmonary bypass (Adapted from Wan et al. 1997)1

6. The release of cytokines may be stimulated by a number of factors, including ischemia-reperfusion, the complement activation, the release of endotoxins and the effect of other cytokines;
7. The platelet-activating factor (PAF) has a crucial role in the lesion of myocardial ischemia-reperfusion and may also have hemodynamic deleterious effects during the CPB;
8. The excessive production of NO, by the expression of iNOS, may be the result of these multiple mechanisms, being the biggest cause of the vasoplegic syndrome;
9. There may be an increase of endothelin levels during the CPB, surgical treatment of congenital cardiopathy, valve disease and CABG. Its role is not clear in the physiopathology of the post-CPB vasoplegia. Otherwise, if the vasoplegia is a consequence of a large release of NO, its opponent vasoconstrictor effect does not manifest.

7.2. Vasopressin-dependent mechanisms

Landry et al. [28] showed that the levels of vasopressin in septic shock are abnormally low. This fact supports the hypothesis that, in sepsis, there may be a decrease in vasopressin stocks and/or a baroreflex dysfunction, causing an insufficient secretion of vasopressin. These authors reported also situations of sepsis with refractory hypotension, which was recovered by the injection of vasopressin that led to a reduction of the needs of catecholamines.

Considering the similarities of the inflammatory response in sepsis and post-CPB vasoplegia, Argenziano et al [29] published a retrospective analysis of 40 cases of distributive shock after heart surgery treated with vasopressin. These same authors included in their experience with this drug the heart transplant and patients who underwent mechanical circulatory assistance. In these patients, there was no hypertensive rebound, peripheral or mesenteric ischemia, closed to an improvement in blood pressure levels and decrease of the needs of catecholamines.

Based on this experience Talbot et al. [30] published the case of a patient who had refractory hypotension at the beginning of the CPB, possibly associated with high levels of potassium cardioplegia and the prolonged use of diuretics and ramiprilat. It was used a unit of vasopressin bolus with immediate pressure response, suspension of catecholamines, and without any observable collateral effect. The efficiency and safety of this new and promising agent pressure needs further observation.

7.2.1. Possible therapeutic strategies

The corticosteroids have been used in heart surgery for more than 30 years attributed to a number of effects: 1) improvement on hemodynamic conditions, 2) lower vasoconstriction with improved tissue perfusion, 3) cellular effects such as stabilization of the lysosome membrane, 4) inhibition of phospholipase A2 activation with stabilization of lipid cell membranes, 5) antiinflammatory activity with lower release of cytokines and inhibition of complement activation and, 6) Selective inhibition of iNOS demonstrated experimentally by the action of dexamethasone.

Although it is use has an experimental and logical basis, many studies failed to demonstrate it is real effectiveness. Some studies try to attribute an anti-inflammatory activity to the aprotinin in situations of ischemia-reperfusion and association with the use of oxygenators with heparinized surface, but the controversial aspects about their concrete effectiveness do not justify its routine use.

Similarly, the use of antioxidants in the preoperative, the use of surface oxygenators with heparinized surface and depletion of leukocytes are also speculative subjects. However, the use of techniques of ultrafiltration and "cell savers" may be considered beneficial because these techniques are employed almost as a routine in American services, where there is the impression that the vasoplegic shock is not considered a serious problem. The removal of proinflammatory substances and the decrease of the contact of white blood cells with the CPB circuit certainly are useful functions of these two techniques [26]. These strategies are represented in Figure 4.

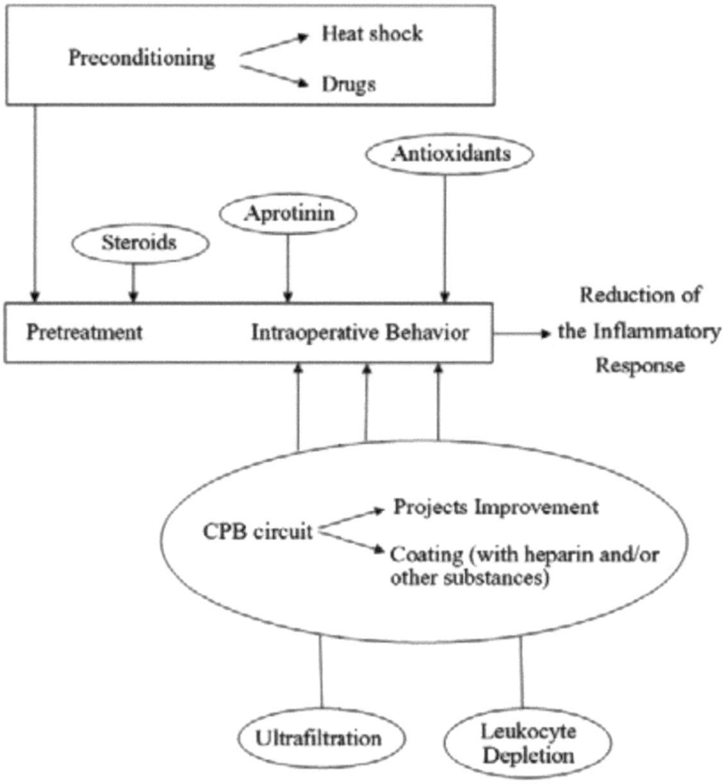

Figure 4. Possible therapeutic strategies to reduce the inflammatory response during cardiopulmonary bypass (Adapted from Wan et al. 1997)

7.3. The inhibition of guanylate cyclase by methylene blue as therapeutic propose for vasoplegia associated to cardiopulmonary bypass

The vasoplegic syndrome associated with the CPB was described by Gomes et al. [31] in 1994 and Evora et al proposed that the vasoplegia was dependent on the cyclic GMP system [32, 33]. In clinical impossibility of NO production from the L-arginine, it was proposed the inhibition of guanylate cyclase by the use of methylene blue. Nowadays, this approach seems to be the most reasonable proposal therapy since it does not interfere with the Nitric Oxide synthesis, and as a medication widely used in other clinical conditions. The action of methylene blue involves at inhibition of the guanylate cyclase avoiding the increase of cyclic GMP and thus avoiding the endothelium-dependent relaxation mediated by NO [34, 35].

Although methylene blue has been used to treat vasoplegic syndrome, over 15 years, there are few human studies to adopt a treatment protocol. Only three studies involving a larger number of patients deserves, due to their importance, the inclusion in this review about CPB [36]. In

2003, Leyh et al. [37] reported 54 cases of cardiac surgical patients with no bacterial endocarditis who were treated with methylene blue with response to the treatment of over 90% of patients. Levin et al. [38] reported incidence of 8.8% of vasoplegic syndrome in 638 patients, with 56 patients randomized to receive vasoplegic methylene blue or placebo.

There were no deaths in the group that used methylene blue and the vasoconstrictor amines could be discontinued in a short time, with consequent lower morbidity and mortality. In the placebo group occurred two deaths, the use of amines lasted around 48 hours with the highest incidence of respiratory and kidney problems. This study supported the idea of methylene blue as efficient treatment of the vasoplegic syndrome.

Regarding to prevention of the vasoplegic syndrome, Ozal et al. [39], in a prospective randomized study showed that methylene blue was associated with a lower incidence of vasoplegia and less use of sympathetic amines. The criterion for inclusion of more patients in the study protocol was (in addition to the use of heparin) the use of ACE inhibitors. These two drugs are, up to now, the only ones considered as a risk factor for vasoplegic syndrome.

Finally, this study may not let to make considerations about the "unanswered question" about the use of methylene blue: Why does the vasoplegic presentation reverse itself promptly sometimes, and occasionally seem not effective? Recently, a brilliant doctoral thesis was defended at the Federal University of Florianopolis (which has already been published by Fernandes et al. [40]) and brings some extraordinarily powerful data to attempt to answer that question. Based on a mice sepsis model, the authors demonstrated that the guanylate cyclase enzyme dynamics allows a "window of opportunity" for the efficiency of methylene blue. In the first eight hours, no longer occurs vasoreactivity not only by the action of amines, but also by the action of nitric oxide donor drugs.

This phase coincides with increased expression of iNOS. Between eight and sixteen hours, the expression of guanylate cyclase gradually cancels itself, probably by excessive production of nitric oxide, and thus in this stage the methylene blue may not act. Later, between sixteen and twenty-four hours, there would be a "de novo" synthesis of guanylate cyclase and the methylene blue may be effective again.

Considering these findings, we start to use the infusion of methylene blue even without an apparent effectiveness, waiting for the "window of opportunity", or that is, for the "de novo" synthesis of guanylate cyclase. One of our diabetic patients, who developed vasoplegic syndrome during the CPB, presented an excellent response to methylene blue but repeated serious vasoplegia in the surgical ICU without response to methylene blue. We maintained infusion of methylene blue associated to high doses of adrenaline and noradrenaline. At the fourth postoperative day, we repeated new endovenous bolus of methylene blue and the response was terrific and on the fifth day no longer was needed for infusion of amines to maintain arterial pressure and the stability of systemic vascular resistance in normal values.

8. Lung and brain perfusion in cardiopulmonary bypass

The pulmonary infusion is temporarily interrupted during the CPB causing ischemia followed by reperfusion lesion. It is known that the blood supply of the lungs performs by means of two different systems: the pulmonary and bronchial circulation. The bronchial circulation irrigates the supported tissue of the lungs with conjunctive tissue, septum and small bronchioles, while the pulmonary capillary circulation is made by the pulmonary artery branches. Connections between the pulmonary and bronchial circulations are particularly valuable in the absence of pulmonary circulation. In long-term, the bronchial circulation may extend and ensure the functions of affected areas [41].

Changes in pulmonary function after CPB is still extremely significant because they are associated with increased morbidity and mortality. Two main mechanisms, the systemic inflammatory response and normothermic ischemic lesion have been implicated by these alterations. To avoid or prevent these alterations, the perfusion of pulmonary artery during the CPB with aortic clamping has been professed [42]. However, the perfusion of the pulmonary arteries during heart surgery with the use of CPB is not an usual and routine practice, even though the concept of ischemia lesion and pulmonary reperfusion is being showed (clinically and experimentally) as responsible for the deleterious effects in the postoperative period.

Some experimental studies have demonstrated that the perfusion maintenance of the pulmonary artery, with or without drugs, has the advantage of improving pulmonary function after CPB [42, 43]. The advantages of the perfusion of the pulmonary trunk were recently demonstrated in a postdoctoral work developed in the Escola Paulista de Medicina - UNIFESP [44].

The possibility of maintenance of ventilation during the CPB improves the respiratory function of patients undergone heart surgery with CPB is controversial. Meanwhile, metanalysis performed with a strategy based on evidence identified nine studies among 187, which when carefully examined showed no evidence favorable to the maintenance of ventilation during the CPB.

That study showed a variety of strategies including ventilation: a) CPAP with positive pressure, 5-15 cmH2O, b) high-frequency ventilation (with 100 resp/min), c) inspired fractions of oxygen from 21 to 100% and, d) bilateral CPB using the lungs to oxygenate the blood during the CPB. Although some small and transitional benefits have been observed with CPAP of 10cmH2O, no clinical benefit for any of ventilatory strategies during the CPB was established. Therefore, ventilation during the CPB may not be considered to improve the respiratory function of postoperative patients undergone heart surgery with CPB [45].

Unlike the pulmonary perfusion during the CPB, the selective brain perfusion has become consensus and may bring additional benefits to hypothermia during aortic surgery. In general, if it is accepted that the continuous perfusion brain promotes better protection brain, its association with hypothermia is still subject of controversy. One of them concerns the initial period of hypothermic cardiac arrest that may negatively affect the late evolution of surgical patients. Experimental evidence seem to demonstrate that the hypothermia does not involve these developments, perhaps by mechanisms of self-regulation of cerebral blood flow which rises along with their adaptation to the metabolic oxygenation [46].

Finally, it would be unfair if we not mention that the content of a class, showed on the Internet provided by Larson, was one of the motivating factors of this review [47].

9. Essential informations

In the conclusion of this critical review, follows some information that we consider essential throughout the text.

- Surgeons must maintain and improve their knowledge about CPB based on the basic fact of maintaining its educational leadership over their team. On the other hand, there is certain tolerance to the CPB apparatus, because the quality of the material ensures large margin of safety for heart operations.
- During CPB, the circulation physiology is fully modified by the introduction of a non pulsatile flow of arterial side opposed to high venous pressure on the venous side of the circulation.
- Together with the SvO2, which is useful patient's metabolic rate during the CPB, the ÄPCO2 can help to fulfill the role in the adequacy of tissue perfusion during surgery. That gradient, perhaps one of the best parameters of tissue perfusion, maybe for lack of knowledge, is rarely used by perfusionists.
- The CPB techniques are clearly divided into protocols for children and protocols for adults. Therefore, among adults, would not be interesting the elaboration of protocols individually? For example, the elderly and diabetics, due to their individual characteristics. Do they not deserve more appropriate protocols?
- What about the systemic inflammatory response, caused by blood exposure to the nonendothelial surface of CPB circuit?. From verification that the inflammatory response is present in patients operated off-pump, the focus changed to the concept that, rather than contact with the CPB circuit, the contact of blood with the operatory wound may be more responsible for the phenomenon of inflammation in CPB.
- Why does the vasoplegic syndrome sometimes reverse itself promptly, and sometimes seem not be effective? Model of sepsis in mice revealed a "window of opportunity" for the efficiency of methylene blue in helping to restore the systemic vascular resistance. This window of opportunity depends on the dynamics of action of guanylate cyclase that by the intense release of NO by action of iNOS "saturates" itself, losing its activity for a few hours when their "de novo" synthesis occur "again"; when the methylene blue becomes effective again. Therefore, perhaps should be a good idea to maintain the infusion of methylene blue, since the "de novo" synthesis of the enzyme occurs between 18 and 24 hours.
- New technologies (impregnated circuits, "retrograde prime, minicircuits of CPB, techniques to minimize the inflammatory reaction") have been "beneficial", "promising", without

becoming unanimity in the face of routine and conventional techniques of CPB. Thus, as already mentioned, we must "persist in our daily faith that the body is incredibly able to resist and mostly often fixes this physiological chaos."

- Alterations in pulmonary function after CPB is a particularly pertinent question because they are associated with increased morbidity and mortality. Two main mechanisms, the systemic inflammatory response and normothermic ischemic injury have been implicated by these alterations. In order to avoid or prevent these alterations, the pulmonary artery perfusion during the CPB with aortic clamping - although not consensual - has been recommended.
- Although some minor and temporary benefits have been observed with CPAP of 10 cmH2O, no clinical benefit for any of ventilatory strategies during the CPB was established. Thus, pulmonary ventilation during the CPB may not be considered improve the postoperative respiratory function of patients undergone on-pump heart surgery.
- Unlike the pulmonary perfusion during the CPB, the selective perfusion brain has become a consensus and may introduce additional benefits to hypothermia during aortic surgery, but its association with hypothermia is still controversial. Experimental evidences seem to show that the initial hypothermia does not compromise this evolution, perhaps by mechanisms of self-regulation of cerebral blood flow which rise along with their metabolic adaptation to the oxygenation. Experimental evidences seem to show that the initial hypothermia does not impair these developments, perhaps by mechanisms of self-regulation of cerebral blood flow, which rise along with its metabolic adaptation to oxygenation.

Author details

Paulo Roberto Barbosa Evora and Alfredo José Rodrigues

Cardiovascular Division, Riberão Preto Faculty, São Paulo University, São Paulo, Brazil

References

[1] De Souza MHL, Elias DO. Fundamentos da circulação extracorpórea. 2ª ed. 2006. Disponível em: http://perfline.com/livro/index.html

[2] Evora PR. CEC: fisiologia e microcirculação. Aula ministrada no 34º Congresso da Sociedade Brasileira de Cirurgia Cardiovascular, Florianópolis; 2007.

[3] Barak M, Katz Y. Microbubbles: pathophysiology and clinical implications Chest. 2005;128(4):2918-32.

[4] de Vroege R, te Meerman F, Eijsman L, Wildevuur WR, Wildevuur CHR, van Oeveren W, et al. Induction and detection of disturbed homeostasis in cardiopulmonary bypass. Perfusion. 2004;19(5):267-76.

[5] Rousou JA, Engelman RM, Flack JE 3rd, Deaton DW, Garb JL, Owen SG. The 'primeless pump': a novel technique for intraoperative blood conservation. Cardiovasc Surg. 1999;7(2):228-35.

[6] Gibbon JH Jr. Application of a mechanical heart and lung apparatus to cardiac surgery. Minn Med. 1954;37(3):171-85.

[7] Panico FG, Neptune WB. A mechanism to eliminate the donor blood prime from the pump-oxygenator. Surg Forum. 1960;10:605-9.

[8] DeBois WJ, Rosengart TK. Retrograde autologous priming reduces blood use. Ann Thorac Surg. 1998;66(3):987-8.

[9] Balachandran S, Cross MH, Karthikeyan S, Mulpur A, Hansbro SD, Hobson P. Retrograde autologous priming of the cardiopulmonary bypass circuit reduces blood transfusion after coronary artery surgery. Ann Thorac Surg. 2002;73(6):1912-8.

[10] Dunn J, Kirsh MM, Harness J, Carroll M, Straker J, Sloan H. Hemodynamic, metabolic, and hematologic effects of pulsatile cardiopulmonary bypass. J Thorac Cardiovasc Surg. 1974;68(1):138-47.

[11] Reis CL, Evora PR, Ribeiro PJ, Brasil JC, Otaviano AG, Bongiovani HL, et al. Fluxo pulsátil em circulação extracorpórea. Apresentação de um sistema mecânico com estudos preliminares hemodinâmicos e do transporte de oxigênio. Arq Bras Cardiol. 1984;43(4):239-44.

[12] Hindman B. Cerebral physiology during cardiopulmonary bypass: pulsatile versus nonpulsatile flow. Adv Pharmacol. 1994;31:607-16.

[13] Perthel M, Kseibi S, Sagebiel F, Alken A, Laas J. Comparison of conventional extracorporeal circulation and minimal extracorporeal circulation with respect to microbubbles and microembolic signals. Perfusion. 2005;20(6):329-33.

[14] Perthel M, El-Ayoubi L, Bendisch A, Laas J, Gerigk M. Clinical advantages of using mini-bypass systems in terms of blood product use, postoperative bleeding and air entrainment: an in vivo clinical perspective. Eur J Cardiothorac Surg. 2007;31(6): 1070-5.

[15] Mangoush O, Purkayastha S, Haj-Yahia S, Kinross J, Hayward M, Bartolozzi F, et al. Heparin-bonded circuits versus nonheparin-bonded circuits: an evaluation of their effect on clinical outcomes. Eur J Cardiothorac Surg. 2007;31(6):1058-69.

[16] Campbell EJ, O'Byrne V, Stratford PW, Quirk I, Vick TA, Wiles MC, et al. Biocompatible surfaces using methacryloylphosphorylcholine laurylmethacrylate copolymer. ASAIO J. 1994;40(3):M853-7..

[17] De Somer F, Francois K, van Oeveren W, Poelaert J, De Wolf D, Ebels T, et al. Phosphorylcholine coating of extracorporeal circuits provides natural protection against blood activation by the material surface. Eur J Cardiothorac Surg. 2000;18(5):602-6.

[18] Deppisch R, Göhl H, Smeby L. Microdomain structure of polymeric surfaces— potential for improving blood treatment procedures. Nephrol Dial Transplant. 1998;13(6):1354-9.

[19] Tonner PH, Kampen J, Scholz J. Pathophysiological changes in the elderly. Best Pract Res Clin Anaesthesiol. 2003;17(2):163-77.

[20] Loran DB, Zwischenberger JB. Thoracic surgery in the elderly. J Am Coll Surg. 2004;199(5):773-84.

[21] Matata BM, Galiñanes M. Cardiopulmonary bypass exacerbates oxidative stress but does not increase proinflammatory cytokine release in patients with diabetes compared with patients without diabetes: regulatory effects of exogenous nitric oxide. J Thorac Cardiovasc Surg. 2000;120(1):1-11.

[22] Matata BM, Galiñanes M. Effect of diabetes on nitric oxide metabolism during cardiac surgery. Diabetes. 2001;50(11):2603-10.

[23] Seghaye MC, Duchateau J, Grabitz RG, Wolff T, Marcus C, Engelhardt W, et al. Effect of sodium nitroprusside on complement activation induced by cardiopulmonary bypass: a clinical and experimental study. J Thorac Cardiovasc Surg. 1996;111(4):882-92.

[24] Shanmugam G. Vasoplegic syndrome: the role of methylene blue. Eur J Cardiothorac Surg. 2005;28(5):705-10.

[25] Pallas F, Larson DF. Cerebral blood flow in the diabetic patient. Perfusion. 1996;11(5): 363-70.

[26] Wan S, LeClerc JL, Vincent JL. Inflammatory response to cardiopulmonary bypass: mechanisms involved and possible therapeutic strategies. Chest. 1997;112(3):676-92.

[27] Myles PS, Leong CK, Currey J. Endogenous nitric oxide and low systemic vascular resistance after cardiopulmonary bypass. J Cardiothorac Vasc Anesth. 1997;11(5): 571-4.

[28] Landry DW, Levin HR, Gallant EM, Seo S, D'Alessandro D, Oz MC, et al. Vasopressin pressor hypersensitivity in vasodilatory septic shock. Crit Care Med. 1997;25(8): 1279-82

[29] Argenziano M, Choudhri AF, Oz Mc, Rose EA, Smith CR, Landry DW. A prospective randomised trial of arginine vasopressin in the treatment of vasodilatory shock after left ventricular assist device placement. Circulation. 1997;96(9 Suppl):II-286-90

[30] Talbot MP, Tremblay I, Denault AY, Bélisle S. Vasopressin for refractory hypotension during cardiopulmonary bypass. J Thorac Cardiovasc Surg. 2000;120(2):401-2.

[31] Gomes WJ, Carvalho AC, Palma JH, Goncalves I Jr, Buffolo E. Vasoplegic syndrome: a new dilemma. J Thorac Cardiovasc Surg. 1994;107(3):942-3.

[32] Andrade JCS, Batista Filho ML, Evora PRB, Tavares JR, Buffolo E, Ribeiro EE, et al. Methylene blue administration in the treatment of the vasoplegic syndrome after cardiac surgery. Rev Bras Cir Cardiovasc. 1996;11(2):107-14.

[33] Évora PR. Should methylene blue be the drug of choice to treat vasoplegias caused by cardiopulmonary bypass and anaphylactic shock? J Thorac Cardiovasc Surg. 2000;119(3):632-4.

[34] Évora PR, Levin RL. Methylene blue as drug of choice for catecholamine-refractory vasoplegia after cardiopulmonary bypass.J Thorac Cardiovasc Surg. 2004;127(3): 895-6.

[35] Évora PR, Viaro F. The guanylyl cyclase inhibition by MB as vasoplegic circulatory shock therapeutical target. Curr Drug Targets. 2006;7(9):1195-204.

[36] Leite EG, Ronald A, Rodrigues AJ, Évora PR. Is methylene blue of benefit in treating adult patients who develop catecholamine-resistant vasoplegic syndrome during cardiac surgery? Interact Cardiovasc Thorac Surg. 2006;5(6):774-8.

[37] Leyh RG, Kofidis T, Strüber M, Fischer S, Knobloch K, Wachsmann B, et al. Methylene blue: the drug of choice for catecholamine-refractory vasoplegia after cardiopulmonary bypass? J Thorac Cardiovasc Surg. 2003;125(6):1426-31.

[38] Levin RL, Degrange MA, Bruno GF, Del Mazo CD, Taborda DJ, Griotti JJ, et al. Methylene blue reduces mortality and morbidity in vasoplegic patients after cardiac surgery. Ann Thorac Surg. 2004;77(2):496-9.

[39] Ozal E, Kuralay E, Yildirim V, Kilic S, Bolcal C, Kücükarslan N, et al. Preoperative methylene blue administration in patients at high risk for vasoplegic syndrome during cardiac surgery. Ann Thorac Surg. 2005;79(5):1615-9.

[40] Fernandes D, Silva-Santos JE, Duma D, Villela CG, Barja-Fidalgo C, Assreuy J. Nitric oxide-dependent reduction in soluble guanylate cyclase functionality accounts for early lipopolysaccharide-induced changes in vascular reactivity. Mol Pharmacol. 2006;69(3):983-90.

[41] Schlensak C, Doenst T, Preusser S, Wunderlich M, Kleinschmidt M, Beyersdorf F. Bronchial artery perfusion during cardiopulmonary bypass does not prevent ischemia of the lung in piglets: assessment of bronchial artery blood flow with fluorescent microspheres. Eur J Cardiothorac Surg. 2001;19(3):326-31.

[42] Liu Y, Wang Q, Zhu X, Liu D, Pan S, Ruan Y, et al. Pulmonary artery perfusion with protective solution reduces lung injury after cardiopulmonary bypass. Ann Thorac Surg. 2000;69(5):1402-7. [Links]

[43] Fan X, Liu Y,Wang Q, YuC, Wei B, Ruan Y.Lung perfusion with clarithromycin ameliorates lung function after cardiopulmonary bypass. Ann Thorac Surg. 2006;81(3): 896-901.

[44] Gabriel EA. Perfusão do tronco pulmonar em cirurgias cardíacas com emprego de circulação extracorpórea [Tese Pós-Doutorado]. São Paulo:Universidade Federal de São Paulo, Escola Paulista de Medicina;2007.

[45] Vohra HA, Levine A, Dunning J. Can ventilation while on cardiopulmonary bypass improve post-operative lung function for patients undergoing cardiac surgery? Interact Cardiovasc Thorac Surg. 2005;4(5):442-6.

[46] Halstead JC, Etz C, Meier DM, Zhang N, Spielvogel D, Weisz D, et al. Perfusing the cold brain: optimal neuroprotection for aortic surgery. Ann Thorac Surg. 2007;84(3): 768-74

[47] Larson DF. Adequacy of perfusion during cardiopulmonary bypass: Empiric or scientific. Disponível em: www.kfshrc.edu.sa/perfusion/education/Perfusion%20Adequacy%20FINAL%202003.

Chapter 3

Hands on as Educational Process in Cardiovascular Surgery

Gilberto Venossi Barbosa,
Carlos Manuel de Almeida Brandão and
Vinicius José da Silva Nina

Additional information is available at the end of the chapter

http://dx.doi.org/10.5772/57113

1. Introduction

Methods of the teaching-learning binomial in cardiovascular surgery has undergone major transformations in the last decade, moving from purely informational content models for environments that stimulate theoretical "know-how" by incorporating skills and competencies [1, 2].

Conducting the training procedures on animal models offers the closest scenario to surgery in human beings; however, the completion of this kind of training requires the sacrifice of these animals culminating with great opposition by the animals' protection organizations as well as by the general population.

This traditional method has well known limitations such as the need for a broad framework for hosting, maintenance and preparation of these animals and their subsequent disposal; which besides of high costs also requires the involvement of many professionals for the correct execution of these tasks. Routinely, these facilities are available only in medical schools and usually with restricted access to their own undergraduate or graduate students.

The task of producing scientific knowledge and validate it through the current methods of evidence-based medicine belongs primarily to the universities, which through its institutes and research laboratories, are prepared for this important and crucial stage of development of medical science.

On the other hand, the medical specialty societies must be in charge for the task of training and retraining the graduates of these educational institutions who completed their residency program or fellowship in thoracic and cardiovascular surgery in order to maintain excellence in their daily practice [3, 4].

In the cognitive domain, the transmission and retention of the essential theoretical knowledge are required and of paramount importance for the judgment and proper handling of each patient.

That part has been widely covered by many mini-courses offered at numerous conferences in many different areas of the specialty, and also through continuing medical education programs carried out by schools and educational institutes created and maintained by the specialty societies and supported by pharmaceutical companies for equipments and instruments in cardiovascular surgery [5, 6].

Simply we could synthesize that surgeons should be prepared not only to know how to say, but essentially how do.

Currently, patients want safer treatments that offer greater efficiency with lower potential risks, less pain and faster recovery to their existential and work activities.

The rapid changes occurring in our specialty with the advent of new procedures with greater potential to contemplate the desires and needs described above, and also the dispute of these new treatment methods among professionals in other related areas, become them imperative to broaden the opportunities for qualification of our surgeons [7].

It seems increasingly clear that these new therapies will not be subject to appropriation of a particular specialty, but, of those professionals who are able to perform them with greater competence, i.e., for those getting better results and enabling to resolve their complications [8].

The formation of Heart Team has immense potential to reduce conflicts of opinion, democratize decisions and benefit patients, but our effective participation in it, still dependent on our skills in the practice of therapeutic acts with competence necessary to continue providing the best results.

The congresses of our specialty has been modified each year to discuss the incorporation of these new technologies by presenting the results of numerous studies well designed and well conducted on searching to validate, to disseminate and to extend their use in the daily practice [9].

Watch an operation, usually a complex case or a new procedure, performed at distance in a specialized center and broadcasted to an audience of the event, offers to the participating surgeons an opportunity to interact with the team that performs the surgery and to learn from them some useful surgical aspects; however, this do not endow observers in developing new skills. Additionally, this format has limitations, including legal matters. The surgical team responsible for the operation is subjected to a stress level above the usual. They cannot repeat tactical maneuvers ever performed by the imperative need to continue the operation. Steps or details which were not clear, even if well explained, cannot be repeated. The operation needs to have its normal course and the patient must not be subjected to additional risks, such as stopping at each step of the procedure to allow controversial debates and opinions.

The traditional video sessions, in which procedures can have their technical details presented and discussed, allowing for pauses or repetitions when necessary, are very instructive in providing opportunities for learning technical and tactical details without putting pressure on the surgical team and not subjecting patients to additional risks. This mode helps to understand how to overcome the difficulties in their implementation and the new ways of executing it. Although it is a very useful and attractive format, it does not provide new psychomotor skills for those attending this activity [10].

Therefore, these creative and innovative ways of transmitting knowledge, as described above, do not directly involve the community of observers in surgical procedures fields. The observer surgeons can even assimilate the steps and various tactical maneuvers essential to the operation; however, these do not give them the ability to implement it.

The annual scientific meetings of the various societies of thoracic and cardiovascular surgery worldwide gather at the same time surgeons with extensive experience and some even honored pioneers in surgical techniques with surgeons in the early learning phase and others with several years of experience in the labor market.

These moments are a unique opportunity for a desirable interaction, in that the more experienced ones can help to qualify this critical mass of professionals eager to learn new knowledge, but also willing to incorporate special technical skills as a basic support for their professional performances.

The Hands-On is a different strategy of teaching and learning because it allows interaction between the Expert (surgeon with recognized expertise and competence) with surgeons in different learning curve phases such as residents, junior surgeons or even those with several years of established surgical practice [11].

It differs from other teaching activities once the trainees are directly involved in the whole procedure by "using their hands". The trainee is incentivized to exercise the observation of all steps of the operation, to perform tactical movements and actions ordered in a logical sequence or may be, to incorporate new skills. All this is happening without urgency of time; and above all, under a qualified, enthusiastic and committed guidance and supervision of an Expert [12].

At the same time that it promotes teaching, it allows for both correction and evaluation of performance inducing satisfaction on trainees by creating a the pleasant sense of mastery of new skills or consolidation of the previous ones that now could be executed with a more refined technique [13].

These new skills will be definitely incorporated by salutary practice of exhaustive repetition that will make them automated. Once after its final registration in the brain centers that integrate knowledge with motor skills, it will emerge automatically when requested, completing the cycle: see-search-understand-perform].

2. Purpose

This strategy of teaching-learning is designed to offer live training on surgical techniques in simulators for the participants of the congresses of the specialty under the supervision of an experienced surgeon (EXPERT).

Primary objectives

- To enjoy the experience of experts attending the event;
- To consolidate technical skills in new procedures;
- To master the technical details in inserting new orthotics and prosthetics devices;
- To obtain efficacy in the performance of a specific procedure, avoiding technical flaws that compromise the short and late-term results;
- To incorporate into the surgeons' daily practice these new skills to benefit their patients.

Secondary objectives

- To extrapolate the knowledge acquired at the event on his/her way to work.
- To recognize which of these therapies will impact on their current and future practice.
- To become familiar with the new devices launched by the industry and with their proper use in patients.
- The Hands-On is very important to participants because constitutes a unique opportunity to watch an experienced and renowned expert to demonstrate step by step details of a particular surgical technique, and at the same time enable them to do it soon afterwards under the supervision of that expert.
- The main benefits for those who participate on the Hands-On are: the acquisition of special skills for the precise execution of new techniques and for those techniques already established as effective, which includes all details for executing them with greater security, and also the knowledge for proper use of new prostheses, surgical tools and suturing threads.

So, after this kind of experience, surgeons return to their workplace with greater knowledge and confidence to run more efficiently their surgical practice in those newly learned specific topics, thus directly benefiting their patients by reducing the risks of these procedures and increasing their safety.

In the last decade we have observed a growing supply of this type of teaching modality in large international congresses. In Brazil Andrade et al in 1993 [14], showed for the first time at an international symposium in Sao Paulo the "Laboratory of Cardiac Surgery", where renowned surgeons performed operations in a simulator located in a glass walls operating room mounted on the amphitheater of the convention center.

The operation was filmed and the images transmitted to a screen displayed in the same amphitheater, allowing interactivity between the surgical team and the participants of the

http://dx.doi.org/10.5772/57113

session. This lab was kept been used for 3 subsequent years in National Congress of the Brazilian Society of Cardiovascular Surgery; however, due to its laborious logistics and high cost it was subsequently discontinued.

In 1986, as a preceptor for medical residency in thoracic and cardiovascular surgery at the Hospital of the Federal University of Rio Grande do Sul in Brazil, we have built a simple simulator, consisting of a wooden shaped-box with an internal structure large enough to fit a porcine or a bovine heart in anatomical position in order to provide a training scenario for the residents in mitral valve surgery.

This model have being used for many years to train several generations of surgeons, whose report thereof, after several years of practice in specialty, convinced us that this was a good and useful strategy with high potential to reduce the learning curve [12].

From this experience, we have designed and developed prototype simulators for valve surgery, coronary artery bypass grafting, correction of atrial fibrillation, cardiac transplantation, repair of congenital heart diseases and for minimally invasive video-assisted cardiac operations named these prototypes as "Professor Barbosa Cardiovascular Simulators".

We have developed three basic models for different purposes but of interchangeable use, characterizing them as low, medium and high fidelity.

In the low-fidelity model the heart not lies in the anatomic position and the area of the intervention is widely exposed facilitating the visualization and manipulation of anatomical structures and the performance of all steps of the procedure without imposing great hardship (Figs. 1).

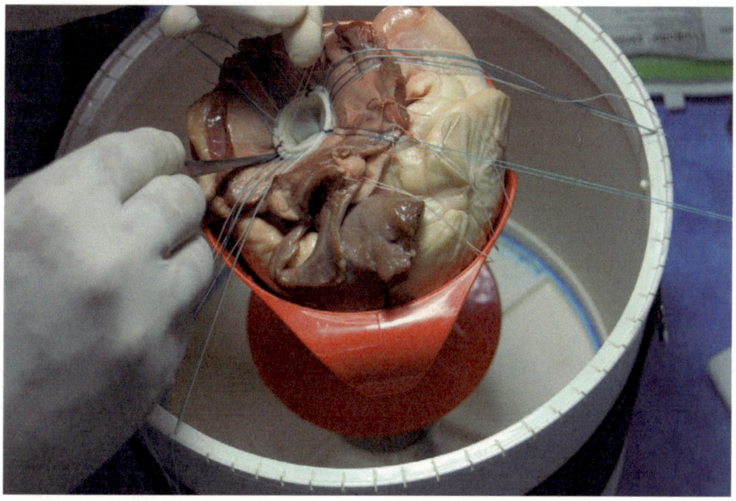

The Medium-fidelity model provides an intermediate degree of difficulty; while in the high-fidelity model the heart is anatomically positioned as well as the structure to be approached on the intervention, mimicking a normal surgical field and offering the same level of difficulty of an intervention on a patient (Figs. 2 and 3).

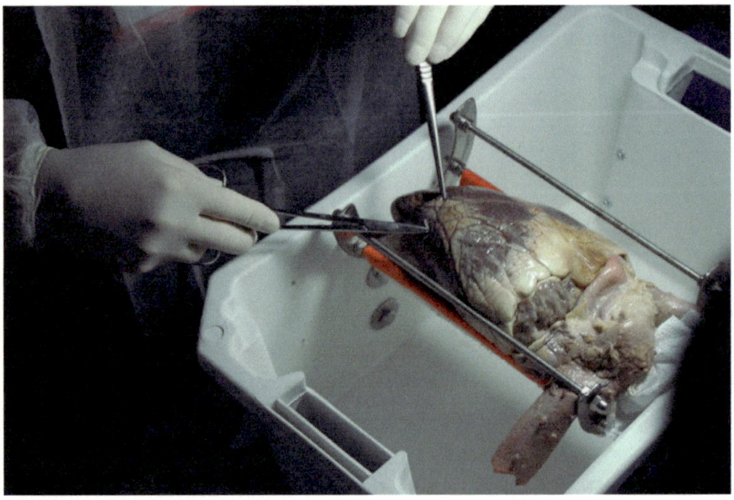

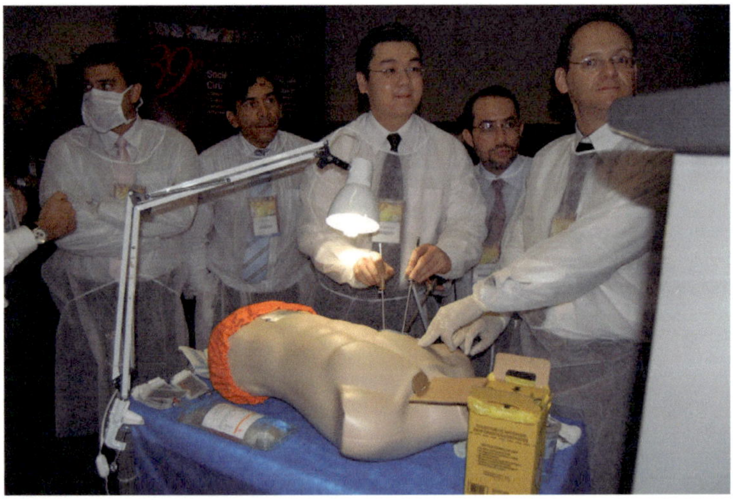

3. General basic features of the simulators

These devices are intended to facilitate the development of specific skills necessary for effective performance in cardiovascular operations, minimizing the required time in the process of learning curve.

It also favors individual or group training on established techniques or new techniques and enables the performance and relationship of a team in systematizing routine procedures or new procedures.

The models have some main constructional features such as the use of lightweight, durable and easy to clean materials making their installation and portability easy, so they can be transported and used in several environments.

The models can harbor either porcine or bovine cardiopulmonary blocs or plastic and polymeric anatomical pieces. The cardiopulmonary blocs are obtained from slaughter houses for human consumption, avoiding the traditional sacrifice of other species in laboratories of experimental surgery (Figs.4 and 5).

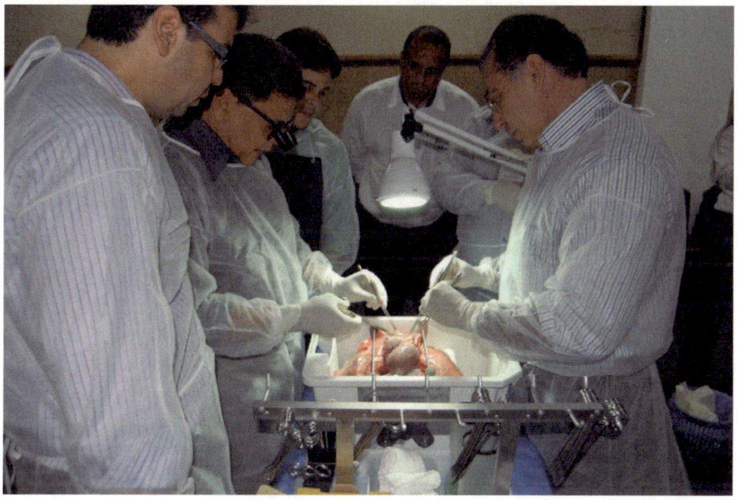

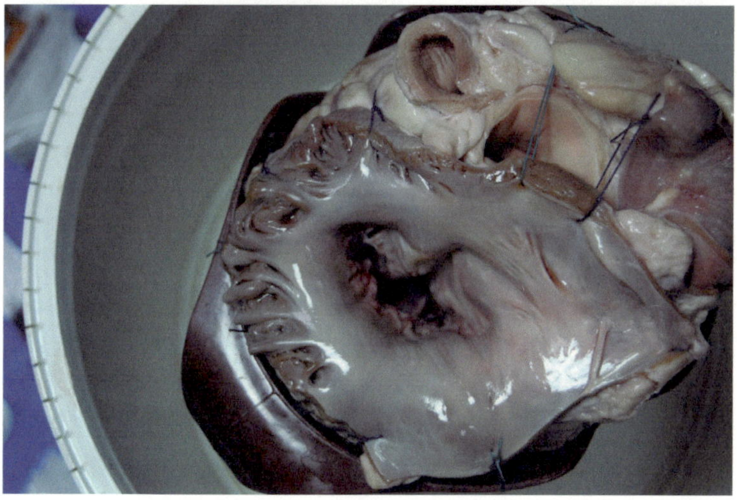

Another advantage of the simulator is that its central part is mobile and deployable allowing that the anatomical structure could to be installed and stored in a freezer getting ready for later use (Figs. 6).

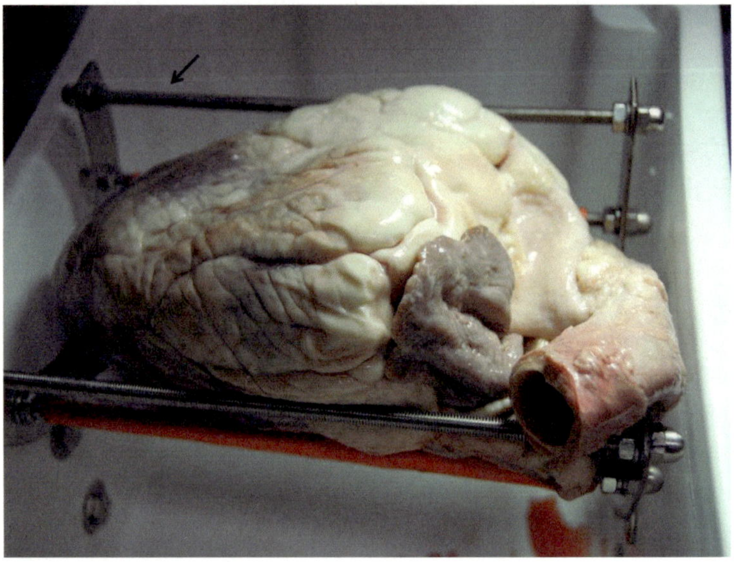

We have also developed an auxiliary unit for orderly displaying the surgical instruments and other materials necessary to perform the operation (Fig. 7).

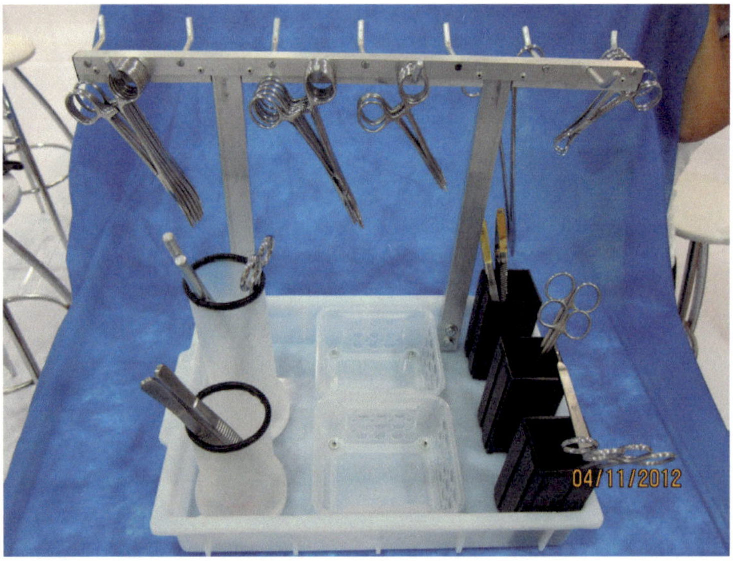

Despite the simplicity of these simulators they have proven effectiveness for their intended purposes, since they can mimic the needs and difficulties experienced during surgery in humans.

As it was necessary to test them more broadly, we have decided to try them during major events to evaluate its effectiveness and gather feedback information from both trainees and experts in order to improve its characteristics.

In the last three annual meetings of the Brazilian Society of Cardiovascular Surgery (2010, 2011, 2012) we have resumed the Hands-On sessions as a priority activity by offering a large volume of sessions and of attendance positions [15, 16, 17].

The use of simulators during these events enabled us to evaluate them and to make changes suggested by the users and also by those derived of our attentive observation serving as the basis for the development of third and fourth generation of prototypes with clear improvement of their performances.

The planning of this activity starts one year prior the meeting and needs a local and national working force so that all details can be planned and discussed with the scientific and executive committee of the congress.

The selection of operations to be inserted on the modules of the Hands-On sessions takes into account their proven efficacy but with still low adoption rates among surgeons, and also new procedures restricted to few centers but in frank expansion in the surgical community worldwide.

As examples we can quote: mitral and tricuspid valvuloplasty, repair of atrial fibrillation, the Ross procedure, and the video-assisted minimally invasive and endovascular procedures and others (Figs. 8, 9, 10, 11 and 12).

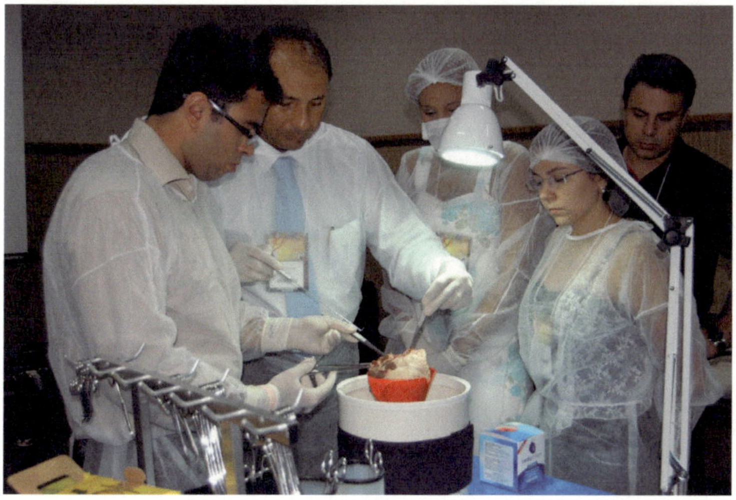

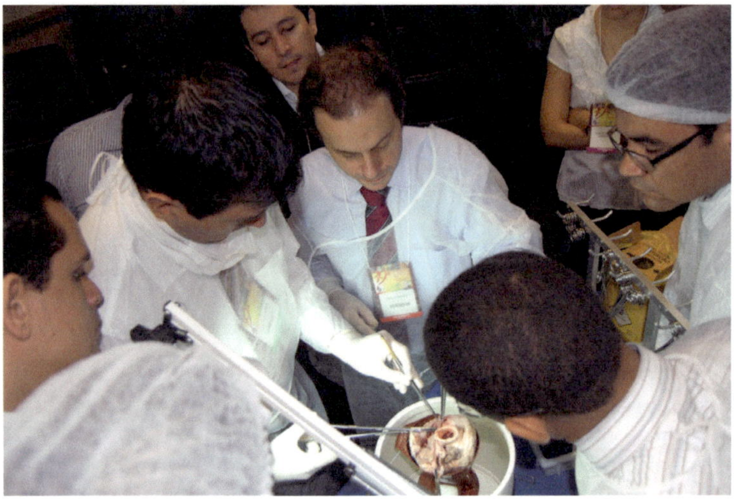

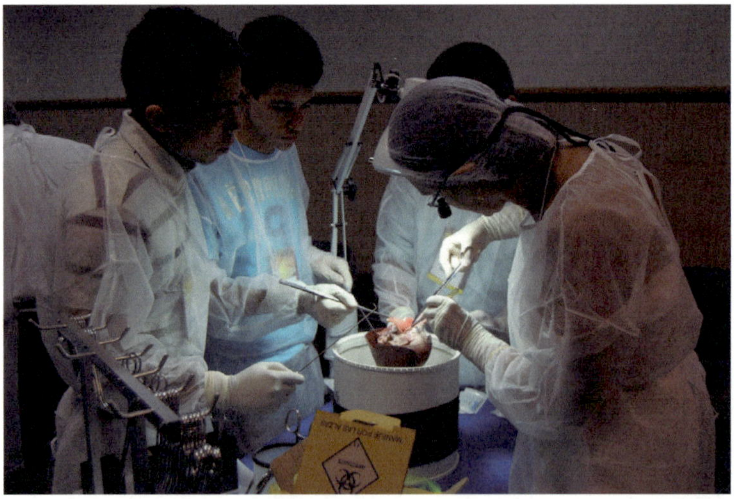

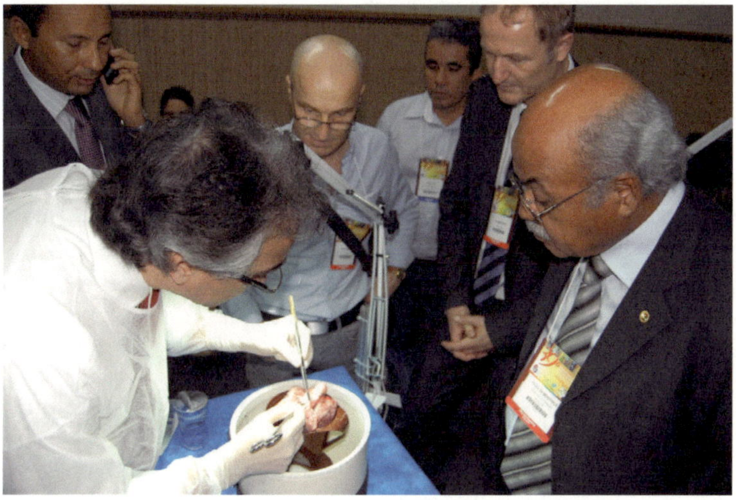

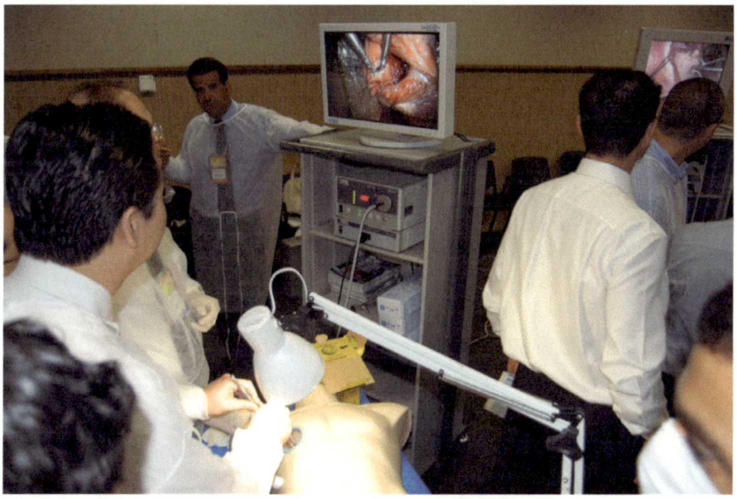

4. Infrastructure facilities and staff

4.1. Room for the setting up the simulators and for the preparation of the anatomical specimens

This room must have minimum dimension of 100 m^2 of area with enough space to house all equipments, materials and working teams, which must also possess an adequate air conditioning system.

Besides of an adequate lighting, the room should have many points of electricity outlets distributed along their walls to connect the equipment and to facilitate the plugging of extension cables, which allow for the installation of lights on the individual working stations.

Equipments:

- Four upright freezers with glass front door with a minimum capacity of 600 liters each, equipped with thermostat and adjustable divisions for storage and maintenance of the anatomical specimens at adequate temperatures. In these freezers it will also be stored anatomical parts already assembled and cataloged on the simulators for prompt use in each session. The progressive thawing and maintenance at optimal temperatures aims to maintain the viability and flexibility of tissues;
- Workbench with 2 to 3 tanks with an independent water supply for washing the anatomical specimens, surgical instruments and other materials;
- A cylinder of compressed air equipped with a valve system to assist in drying the surgical instruments and other materials;
- An ultrasound washing system for the surgical instruments;
- Three tables with dimensions of approximately 1.0 x 4.0 x 0.80 meters (width x length x height) for the preparation of anatomical specimens and for the insertion and fixation of them on the mobile parts of the simulators. One of this table is intended to set up the instrumentation units for displaying surgical instruments, sutures, surgical towels and other materials;
- Chairs with high-backed seats in adequate numbers to accommodate all members of the working teams and the surgeons responsible for the preparation of anatomical specimens and simulators;
- Five tables located along the walls of the room, with approximate dimensions described above, for receiving the packed boxes containing all materials including: simulators, instrumentation units, surgical instruments, light bulbs, gowns, gloves, sutures, prostheses and other inputs. In this site materials are unpacked and distributed to the desktops;
- Containers for disposal of biological materials, organic waste baskets and disposable items basket.

5. Work team

The SBCCV (Brazilian Society of Cardiovascular Surgery) has a permanent National Committee composed by three (Full Members) cardiovascular surgeons that are responsible for the whole organization and improvement of this activity. This committee elects the procedures to be performed and the experts who will present the techniques to the surgeons during the training. This program is submitted to SBCCV Scientific Board for approval.

http://dx.doi.org/10.5772/57113

Local Committee: composed by one coordinator and at least five members (cardiovascular surgeons) from the state in which the Congress will be realized. This committee is responsible for the selection and storage of the anatomic specimens, according to National Committee rules.

Support Staff: composed by residents in cardiovascular surgery and invited cardiovascular surgeons. This group is responsible for preparing the anatomic specimens to be used in the simulators.

Technical Staff: composed by one nurse (or scrub-nurse) and at least three assistants with experience on operation rooms. This staff is responsible for the cleaning and storage of surgical instruments in the Hands-on Preparation Room, preparation of the work stations, disposal of the used anatomic specimens, cleaning of the Hands-on room.

Administration Staff: one secretary responsible for the Hands-on Preparation Room, the surgical instruments, equipments, communication and coordination of the technical staff.

These professionals must work specifically in the Hands-on Program and are coordinated by the National Committee. (Fig. 13)

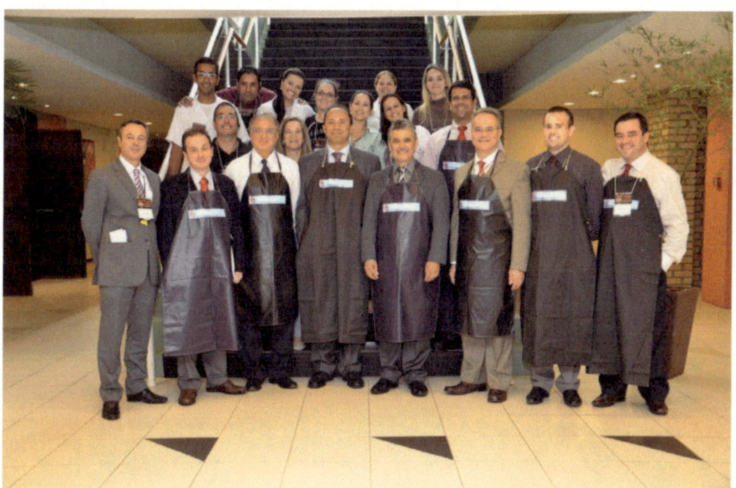

6. Hands-on logistics

The Hands-on Room must support 4 or 5 "work stations", corresponding to a dimension between 70 and 80 m^2. The room must be preferentially rectangular (for instance: 8 X 10 meters), because this configuration allows the free circulation of the participants, technical staff and organizers. The room must have an auxiliary table (for instance: 0.6 X 1.5 meters) to organize the material in use during the procedures (Figs. 14).

The Hands-on Room must have Multimedia Equipment (Computer, Projection, Microphones) for the presentation of the procedures by the "experts" (Figs. 15, 16 and 17).

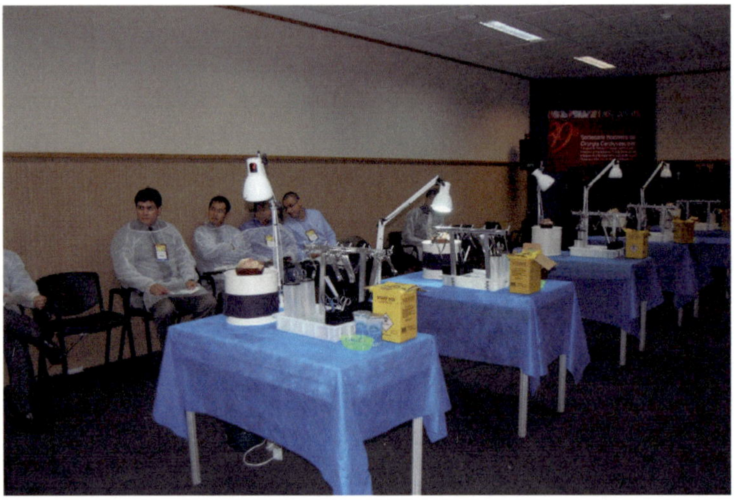

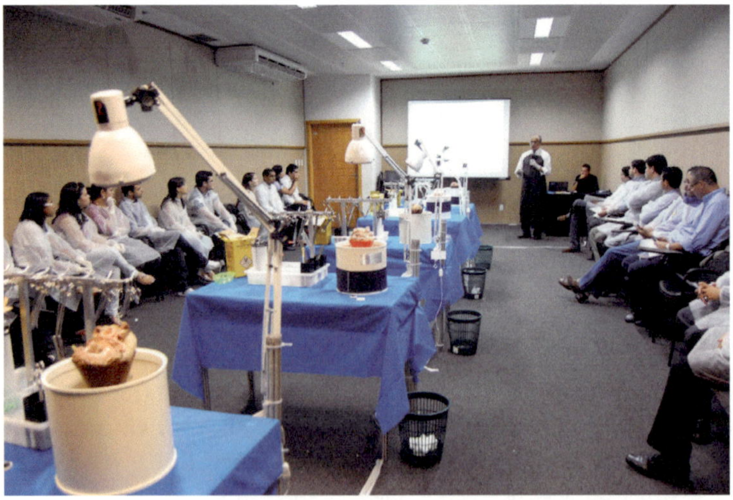

http://dx.doi.org/10.5772/57113

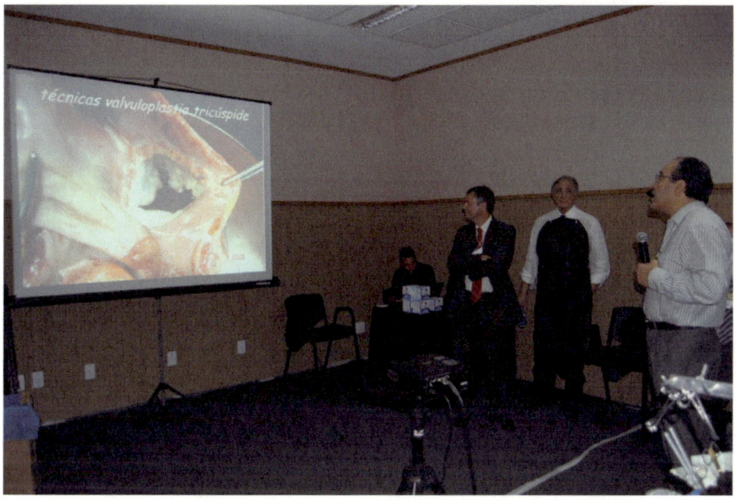

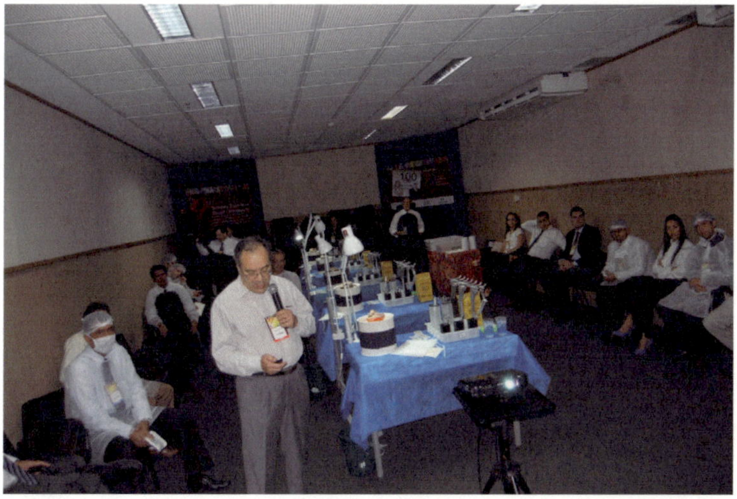

The "Gold Standard" Hands-on is that composed by 4 or 5 rooms, each one with 4 or 5 "work-stations", working simultaneously.

6.1. "Work- stations"

The "work-station" consists in a table with dimensions of 1.2 X 0.6 X 0.8 (length X width X height) meters. The surgical instruments, the simulators with the surgical specimens and all the materials are disposed on these tables (Fig. 18).

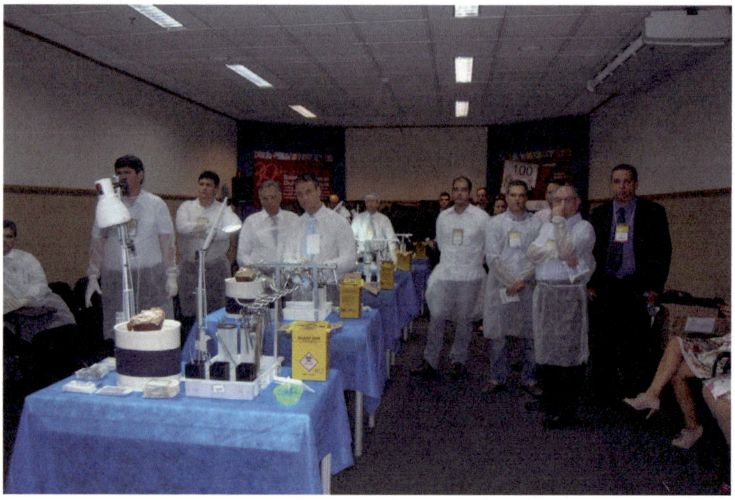

The Expert presents the surgical techniques in the simulators to 3 surgeons, previously registered in the hands-on activity, who will assist the expert first. After the presentation of the surgical technique, these surgeons will perform the procedure with the expert orientation. To repeat the procedure, the technical staff must only remove the central part of the simulator, which contains the surgical specimen, and replace it for another one previously prepared in the "preparation room" (Figs. 19 and 20).

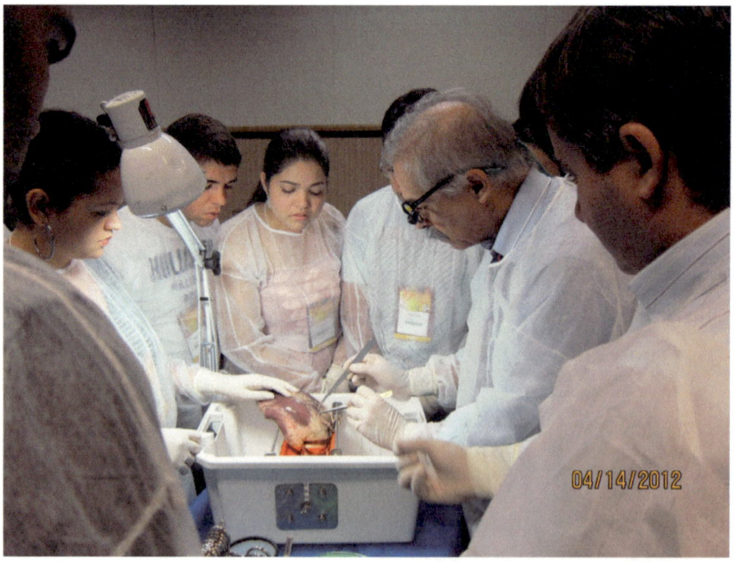

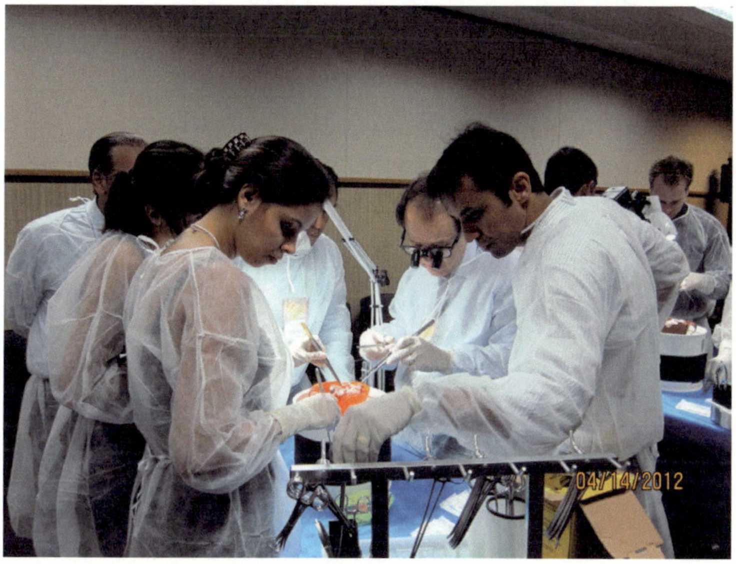

To perform Endovascular or Minimally Invasive Procedures, there must be a larger room, in order to place all the materials used in these procedures.

6.2. Operational steps

1st Step: Registration

The Registration must be preferentially on-line, before the meeting. The Organizing Committee must allow on-site registration only for the remaining places.

The registered participants must receive the information material with the instructions for the Hands-on activity previously.

2nd Step: Room access

There must be a receptionist in each Hands-on room, in order to check the inscriptions and locate the participants in the corresponding "work-station".

3rd Step: Surgical Technique Presentation

The Expert exposes the surgical technique in a short presentation (between 7 and 10 minutes).

4th Step: Hands-on

The Expert presents the surgical techniques in the simulators assisted by the participants. After the presentation of the surgical technique, these surgeons will perform the procedure with the expert orientation.

5th Step: Cleaning

After the procedures, the technical and support (residents) staff removes the surgical specimens, waste material (gloves, sutures, etc) and prepares the simulators for the next session. This step takes between 10 and 15 minutes.

6th Step: Surgical Instruments and Simulators Removal

After the last session of the day, the technical and support staff removes all the surgical instruments and simulators in order to clean it. The room must also be cleaned for the next day.

7th Step: Preparation of the next day Hands-on

After cleaning the room and the instruments, the "work-stations" must be prepared again for the next day activities.

The National Committee and the Local Committee must check all these steps, in order to perform the Hands-on activity on schedule.

6.3. Experience of the Brazilian Society of Cardiovascular Surgery (SBCCV)

In the last 3 SBCCV Congresses, the Hands-on activity was in evidence. It was carried out during 2 days, with 4 sessions a day, each session composed by 3 different wet labs, performing 24 wet labs each Congress. The wet labs have a duration time of 2 hours and each one included 4 work- stations, performing 288 work-stations during the Congress period [15, 16, 17].

Attendees in the Hands-on activities were 864 participants. From these, 62% were previously registered on-line in the Congress website. 288 expert surgeons were invited by the National Committee and the Scientific Board during these activities, many of them international guests (Figs. 21 and 22) and others are national guests (Figs. 23, 24 and 25).

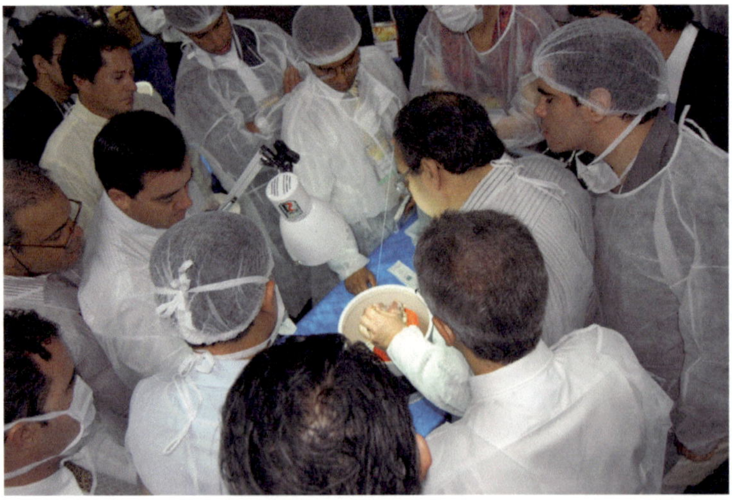

http://dx.doi.org/10.5772/57113

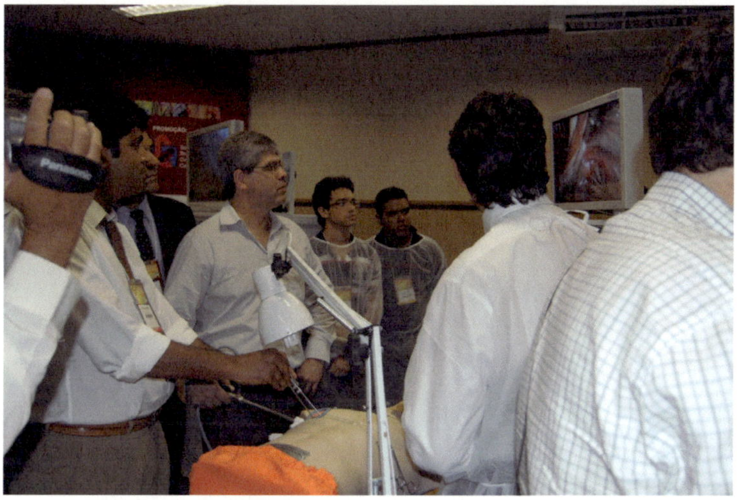

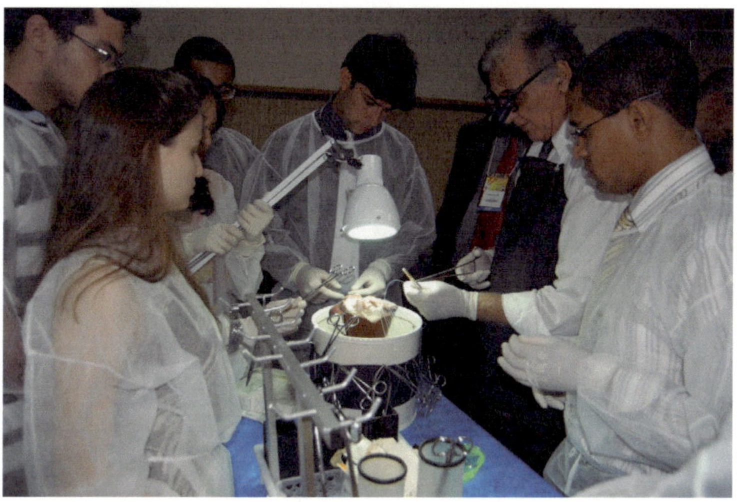

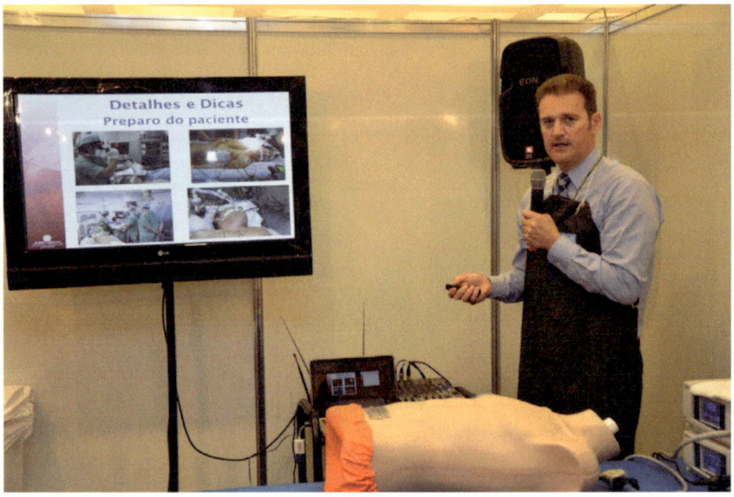
Detalhes e Dicas
Preparo do paciente

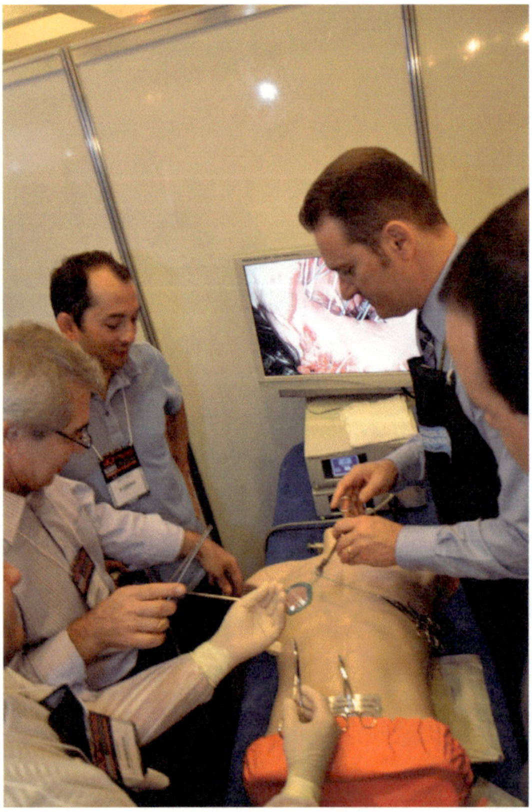

Including the participants, 1152 cardiovascular surgeons were included in the Hands-on activities, what represents the greatest number of surgeons that performed Hands-on activities in International Congresses, according to the present literature (Figs. 26 and 27).

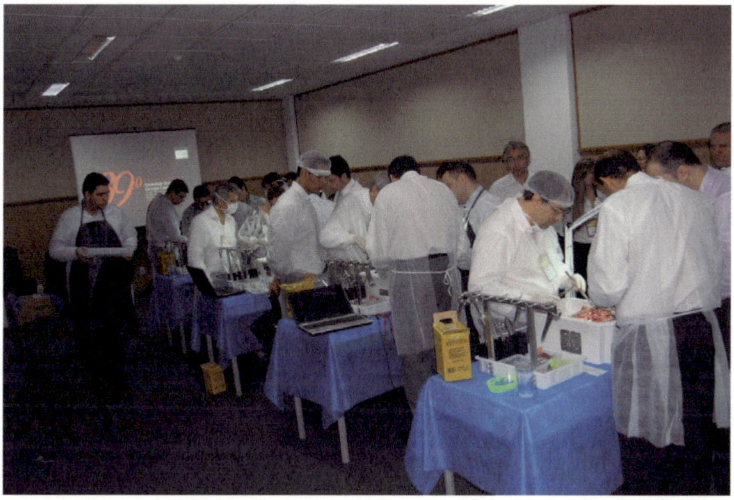

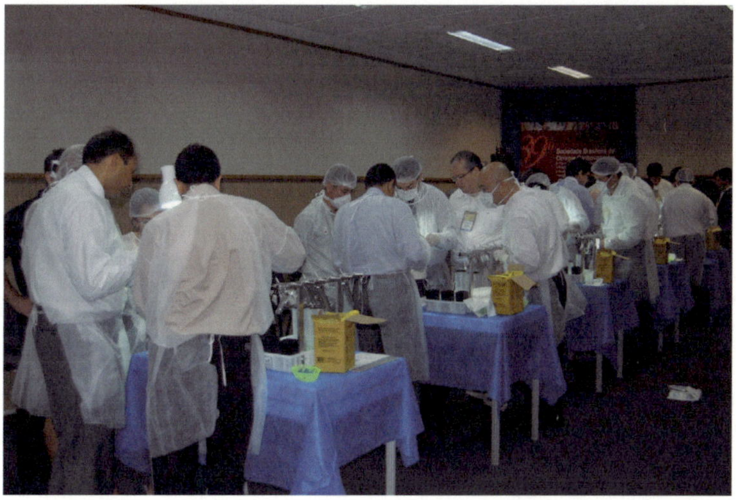

The evaluation forms reported by 76% of the participants, showed a massive approval of this activity in our Congress.

The SBCCV and their 9 Regional Societies performs Hands-on activities in their Regional Congresses and Meetings all over Brazil during the last decade.

In conclusion, we think that these Hands-on activities must be available in all the events of our specialty, once this method of "watching-doing", offers the opportunity of training new technologies and new surgical techniques, and also that these activities must be coordinated by an efficient Committee. The routine implementation of this strategy by each cardiovascular team in their workplace, become a potential tool to reduce the learning curve and increasing the patients safety.

Author details

Gilberto Venossi Barbosa[1,2], Carlos Manuel de Almeida Brandão[2,3] and Vinicius José da Silva Nina[2,4,5]

1 Department of Surgery of the School of Medicine, Universidade Federal do Rio Grande do Sul, Brasil

2 Brazilian Society of Cardiovascular Surgery, Brasil

3 Instituto do Coração (INCOR) do Hospital de Clinicas da Universidade de São Paulo, Brasil

4 Department of Surgery of the School of Medicine, Universidade Federal do Maranhãol, Brazil

5 University Hospital da Universidade Federal do Maranhão, Brasil

References

[1] O'Reagan JD. Leonardo Da Vinci Award for training excelence. Eur J Cardiothorac Surg 2012;41:986-987.

[2] Lodge D, Grantcharov. Training and assessment of technical skills and competency in cardiac surgery. Eur J Cardiothorac Surg 2001;39: 287-94.

[3] Carpentier AJ, Yang SC, Ughlig PN, Colson YL. Envisioning simulation in the future of thoracic surgical education. J Thorac Cardiovasc Surg. 2008;135:477-84.

[4] Ericsson KA. Deliberate practice and acquisition of expert performance: a general overview. Acad Emerg Med.2008;15;988-94.

[5] Antunes M, El Khoury G, Kolh P. Adult Cardiac Surgery Postgraduate Course. In: Proceedings book published by European Association For Cardio-Thoracic Surgery, 21 st Annual Meeting of the European Association For Cardio-Thoracic Surgery, 15-19 September 2007, Geneve Switzerland: Congress Centre.

[6] Pomar JL. Adult Cardiac Surgery Posgraduate Course. In: Proceedings book published by European Association For Cardio-Thoracic Surgery, 23rd Annual meeting of

European Association For Cardio-Thoracic Surgery, 17-21 October 2009, Vienna, Áustria: Austria Centre Vienna

[7] Papaspyros S, Javangula KC, O'Regan DJ. Surgical training in the 48h week: a novel simulation and educational tool. From amateur golfer to Professional pilot. Eur J Cardiothorac Surg 2009;36:511-6.

[8] Raemer DB. Simulation in cardiothoracic surgery: A paradigm shift in education? J Thorac Cardiovasc Surg.2009;138; 1065-1066.

[9] Prenger KB, De Paulis R. Wet Lab training - advanced techniques in cardiac surgery. In: ICVTS 2010;11 (Suppl 2):xxxvi. 24th Annual Meeting of the European Association for Cardio-Thoracic Surgery, 11-15 september 2010, Geneva, Switzerland: Convention Centre.

[10] Pomar JL, Alfieri O, Falk V, Pepper J. Acquired Cardiac Disease Posgraduate Course. In: Abstracts ICVTS 2011;13 (Suppl.2) viii. 25 th Annual Meeting of the European Associaton for Cardio-Thoracic Surgery, 1-5 October 2011, Lisbon, Portugal:Lisbon Congress Centre.

[11] Feins RH.Expert commentary: cardiothoracic surgical simulation. J Thorac Cardiovasc Surg. 2008;135:485-6.

[12] Kneebone R.Simulation in surgical training: educational issues and practical implications. Med Educ 2003;37(3):267-777.

[13] Champion HR, Gallager AG.Surgical simulation- à good idea whose time hás come '.BR J Surg 2003;90(7):767-8.

[14] Andrade JCS. A new methodology for teaching and rehearsing of operative techniques in cardiac surgery. Rev Bras Cir Cardiovasc. 1994; 9 (1):1-21.

[15] Barbosa GV, Brandão CMA, Nina JSV, Brandão CMA. Hands On. In: Abastracts Brazilian J Cardiovasc Surg 2010;25 (1 Suppl.1): 28s. 37° Congresso da Sociedade Brasileira de Cirurgia Cardiovascular, 25-27 Março 2010, Belém, Pará: Hangar Centro de Convenções da Amazônia.

[16] Barbosa GV, Brandão CMA, Nina JSV, Brandão CMA. Hands On. In: Abstracts Brazilian J Cardiovasc Surg 2011;26 (1 Suppl.1): 44s. 38° Congresso da Sociedade Brasileira de Cirurgia Cardiovascular, 31 Março - 2 Abril 2011, Porto Alegre, Rio Grande do Sul: Centro de Eventos da PUC-RS.

[17] Barbosa GV, Brandão CMA, Nina JSV, Brandão CMA. Hands On. In: Abstracts Brazilian J Cardiovasc Surg 2012;27 (1 Suppl.1) 37s. 39° Congresso da Sociedade Brasileira de Cirurgia Cardiovascular, 12-14 Abril 2012, Maceió, Alagoas: Centro de Convenções de Maceió.

Chapter 4

Conservative Management of Mitral Insufficiency — An Alternative Approach

Francisco Gregori Junior

Additional information is available at the end of the chapter

http://dx.doi.org/10.5772/57114

1. Introduction

Conservative management of mitral insufficiency is an alternative technique with attractive features. Among the many advocates of valve repair, Alain Carpentier is the best known [1] His techniques include a combination of ring annuloplasty, resection of segments of valve leaflets, and shortening, transposition and sectioning of chordae. However, despite this repertoire of repair maneuvers, replacement of the mitral valve is the most common method used for patients with mitral insufficiency.

Mitral insufficiency (MI), defined as blood regurgitation from the left ventricle to the left atrium through the valve, is a situation predisposing to left ventricular dysfunction, increase of the left atrium, and atrial arrhythmias, regardless of the ethiology. MI is a common feature in rheumatic disease and fibroelastic degeneration. Mitral valve prolapse identified by redundancy of the anterior and/or posterior leaflet, papillary muscle dysfunction, and chordae tendineae elongation or rupture may evolve to mitral insufficiency. Mitral valvuloplasty is an elective procedure for repair of MI, with better results than mitral valve replacement (Akins et al, 1994) [2]

We have employed mitral reconstructive surgery in our Service since 1979 according to Carpentier techniques. We introduced new alternative techniques that have been used in parallel to those traditional procedures.

1.2. Repair of elongated chordae tendineae

In 1989 we introduced a new technique for shortening of elongated chordae tendineae [3]. It is particularly suitable for shortening the chordae tendineae in patients in whom the papillary muscles are either thin or deeper than usual. The shortening performed above the anterior leaflet of the mitral valve, is quite feasible because of the accessible surgical site and easy quantification of the elongation of the chordae tendineae to be corrected.

Once the elongated chordae were identified, the anterior leaflet is exposed and an orifice about two to three millimeters wide is made near the insertion of the elongated chordae (Fig. 1). After that procedure, the elongated chordae is pulled through the orifice with a nerve tractor or even a thick cotton thread so that the anterior leaflet is towered to an appropriate level, resulting in a satisfactory coaptation of the leaflets. The orifice is sutured with interrupted 5-0 polypropylene sutures. The sutures also fasten the chordae to the atrial surface of the anterior leaflet of the mitral valve.

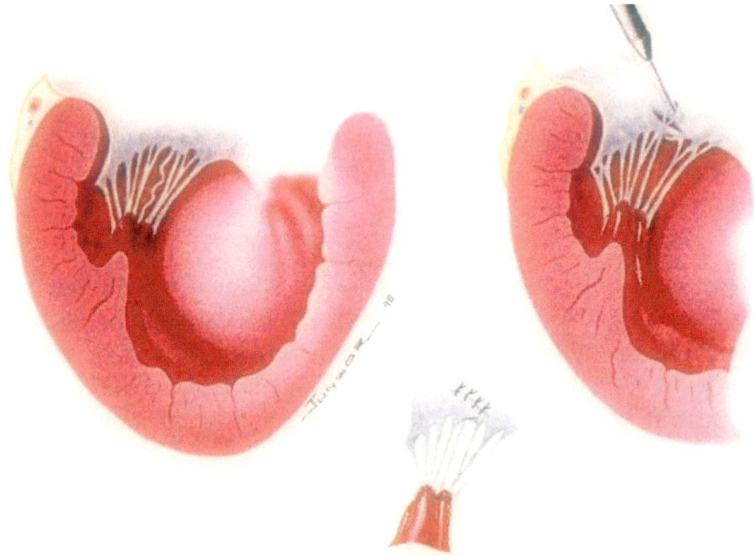

Figure 1. Left - Schematic illustration shows the elongated chorda. Right - Note that the orifice (2 to 3 millimeters wide) is near the edge of the leaflet, at a site corresponding to the insertion site of the elongated chordae. Traction of an elongated chordae through the orifice in the anterior leaflet is observed. The orifice in the anterior leaflet is sutured with interrupted 5-0 polypropylene sutures. Lower - The chordae tendineae are fastened to the atrial surface of the mitral valve.

1.3. Repair of ruptured chordae tendineae

1.3.1. Neo chordae construction [4]

The mitral valve is carefully evaluated and the ruptured or "missing" chordae of the anterior leaflet are located precisely and marked with a suture. Two parallel incisions are made about five to 12 millimeters apart beginning at or near the annulus and carried toward the reference suture up to a point five millimeters from the free border of the leaflet. This strip of tissue thus created is detached beginning near the annulus and is tucked through the slit under the free border, whichever is easier, and brought toward the ventricular cavity. The anterior leaflet is then repaired with interrupted 5-0, polypropylene sutures. The strip is next sutured to the anterior papillary muscle with 5-0 polypropylene mattress sutures. (Fig. 2)

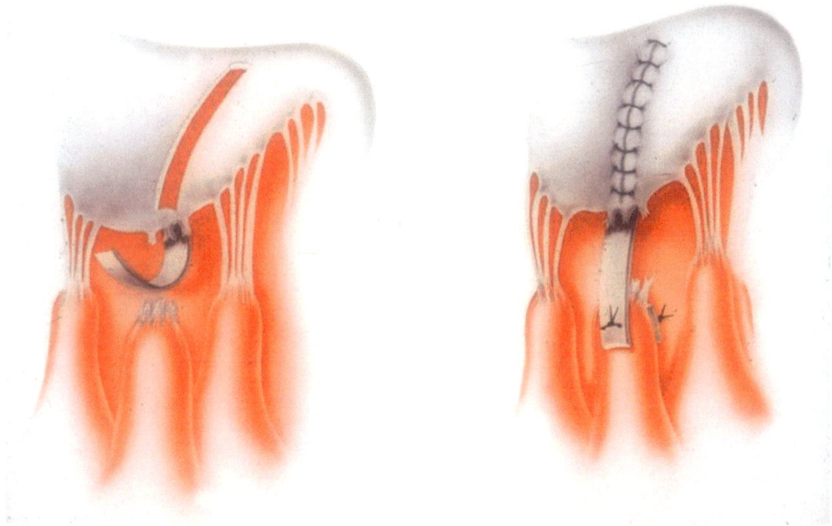

Figure 2. Left - The strip of tissue is tucked through the slit under the edge of the leaflet. Right - The opening in the anterior leaflet is repaired with interrupted 5-0 polypropylene suture and the neochorda is sutured to the anterior papillary muscle with 5-0 mattress sutures.

2. Partial tricuspid valve transfer [5]

Supply of chordae for the anterior leaflet of the mitral valve proceeds according to two techniques. The first and more frequent consists of removal of the posterior leaflet of the tricuspid valve of the patient, with all its elements, that is, with chordae and papillary muscle (Fig. 3). The specimen is transferred to the mitral valve by suturing the papillary muscle to that of the mitral valve, corresponding to the ruptured chordae, using one stitche in U anchored on small Dacron pledgets. After attaching the papillary muscle, the donor leaflet is sutured to the anterior leaflet of the mitral valve avoiding too long chordae, that would cause leaflet prolapse and consequent mitral insufficiency. The same care must be taken with regard to the opposite, that is, chordae retraction with unwanted coaptation of the anterior leaflet causing mitral insufficiency (Fig. 4). The grafted leaflet may be sectioned in the middle, remaining with two heads linked to the papillary muscle by a good number of chordae. One of these heads is sutured to the anterior leaflet and the other to the posterior on (Fig. 5). The tricuspid annulus is plicated with 4-0 polypropylene sutures, anchored on Dacron pledgets at the posterior portion, leaving the bicuspid valve, furthermore correcting any eventual functional tricuspid insufficiency.

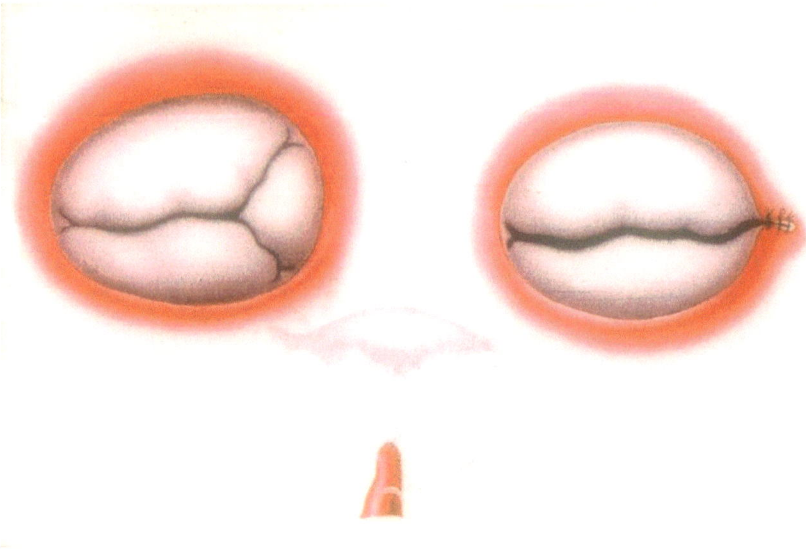

Figure 3. Removal of the posterior leaflet of the tricuspid valve, rendering it bicuspid. The specimen (lower) containing the leaflet, chordae tendineae, and the papillary muscle will be transferred to the mitral valve.

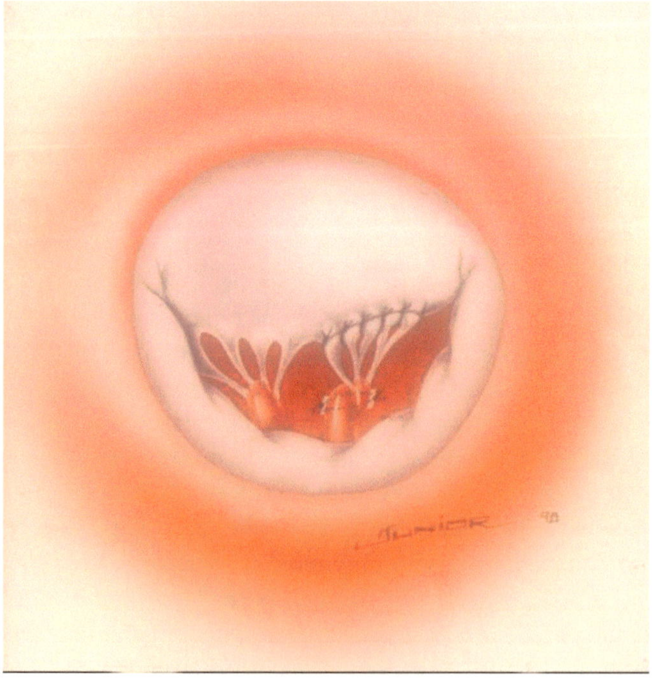

Figure 4. Intraoperative aspect after suture of the graft on the papillary muscle and the anterior leaflet of the mitral valve.

http://dx.doi.org/10.5772/57114

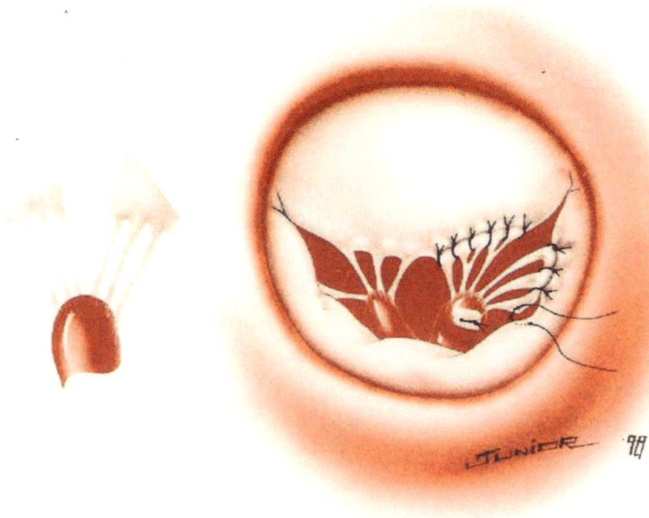

Figure 5. The graft sectioned in the middle remaining with two heads linked to the papillary muscle by a good number of chordae. One head is sutured to the anterior leaflet and the other head to the posterior on.

The second technique (Fig. 6) a variant of the first, is applied when the posterior leaflet of the tricuspid valve, or even the corresponding papillary muscle, were not anatomically adequate. In these cases, the anterior valve is always more developed, to compensate for the small posterior leaflet. Thus, a triangular patch is removed from the anterior leaflet, with a satisfactory number and texture of chordae, and a wedge of the corresponding papillary muscle, wich is transferred to the mitral valve and sutured, likewise to the already described technique. The tricuspid valve in these cases, remains with its three leaflets with the sectioned edges of the anterior leaflet being joined with separated 5-0 polypropylene stitches.

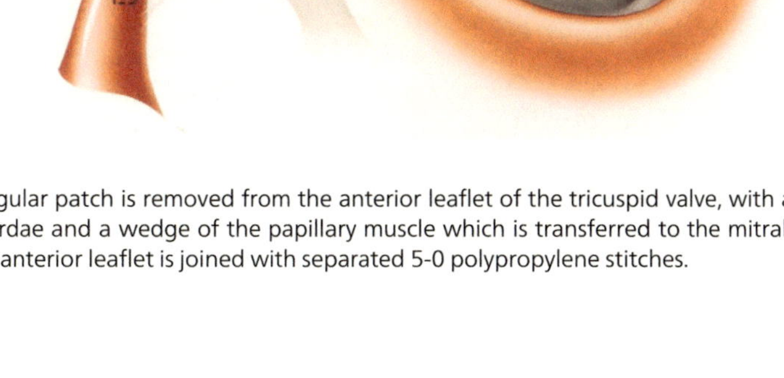

Figure 6. Left - A triangular patch is removed from the anterior leaflet of the tricuspid valve, with a satisfactory number and texture of chordae and a wedge of the papillary muscle which is transferred to the mitral valve. Right – The sectioned edges of the anterior leaflet is joined with separated 5-0 polypropylene stitches.

3. Repair of ruptured chordae or thin elongated chordae by premolded bovine pericardium chords [6]

3.1. The Braile-Gregori prosthesis

The Braile-Gregori Prosthesis (Gregori et al, 1994) [9] created for repair of ruptured chordae is fashioned as a monobloc (Braile Biomédica Industria, Comércio e Representações S/A® – São Paulo – Brazil) joined at their extremities by two polyester-reinforced strips. The standardized bovine pericardium chordae were two millimeters wide and three millimeters distant from each other (Fig. 7) Standardization of the chordae is confirmed by using measuring instruments ranging in length from 20 to 35 millimeters (Fig. 8) The bovine pericardium is treated with 0.5% glutaraldehyde, subjected to anticalcification treatment with glutamic acid, and preserved in 4% formaldehyde solution. Resistance and durability tests showed rupture levels of approximately 15 kg/cm3 (Braile et al, 1990) [7]. The chordae length is determined based on the distance from the top of the papillary muscle to the edge of the leaflet in its original nonprolapsed position.

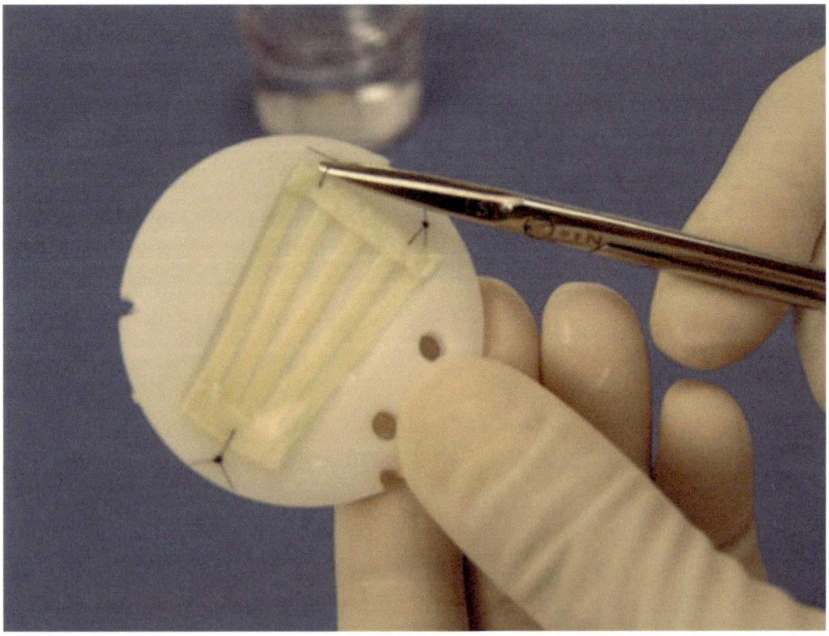

Figure 7. Standardized bovine pericardium chordae.

3.2. The implantation of the prosthesis

The implantation procedure began with anchoring of the prosthesis on the top end of the papillary muscle associated with the ruptured chordae, using one or two 5-0 polypropylene threads anchored in a Dacron pad. Subsequently, the other end is attached, using individual

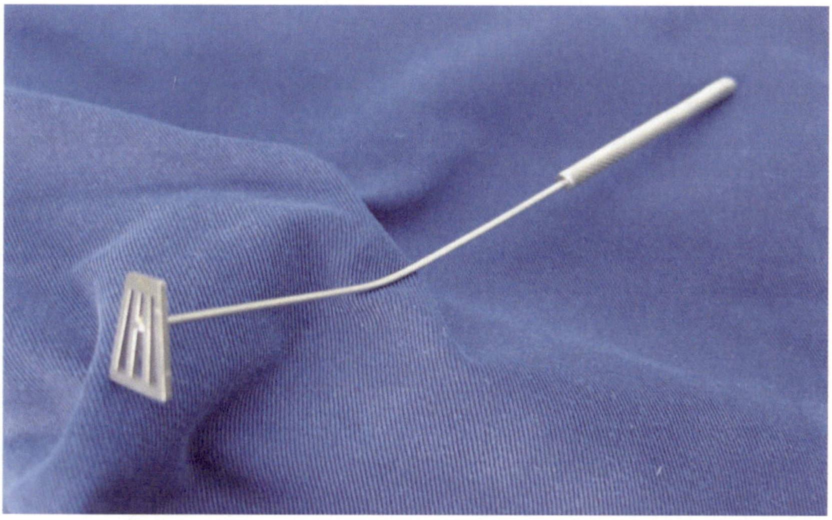

Figure 8. Measuring instruments ranging in length from 20 to 35 mm are used to confirm standardization of the chordae.

5-0 polypropylene sutures, to the free edge of the affected leaflet (Fig 9). The prosthesis, with five standardized chordae, may be reduced to as few as two chordae, as required.

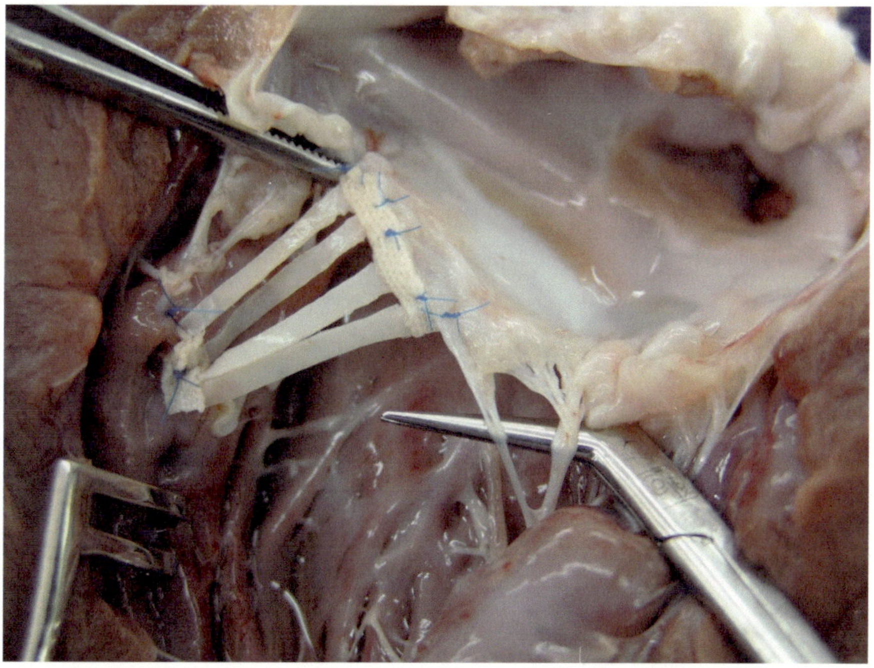

Figure 9. Anatomical aspect of the implantation of the prosthesis in an opened bovine left ventricle.

4. Mitral annuloplasty (gregori-braile ring) [9]

Since the introduction of open valve surgery, annular dilation found in all cases of mitral insufficiency has been treated conservatively. Many Centres, almost simultaneously started correcting mitral insufficiency using plication mitral annuloplasty, a surgical procedure still used today. After having observed anatomic alterations in patients with mitral insufficiency, Carpentier [1] described several techniques for the correction of mitral insufficiency including annuloplasty with a prosthetic ring. Since then, several Centres worldwide have adopted his techniques with excellent results.From 1979 to 1986, we operated on more than 100 patients using Carpentier ring annuloplasty, one-third being under sixteen. Dilation of the anterior side of the mitral annulus between the two fibrous trigonae was demonstrated by Hueb, Jatene and colleagues (2002) [8]. However, it was frequently found posteriorly and to a greater extent posteriorly and next to the postero-medial commissure (Fig. 10). Based on these findings, we developed a semi-circular rigid prosthetic ring (stainless steel wrapped in a thin layer of silicon rubber and covered with Dacron velvet) (Figs.11, 12) with adjustment on its right side, thus correcting the dilation of the posterior side of the mitral ring, next to the postero-medial commissure. The prosthesis corrects the annular dilation (Fig.13) and avoid the late manifestation of mitral stenosis in children and young patients, which is secondary to restraining the normal growth of the mitral ring and observed when closed prosthetic rings are used.

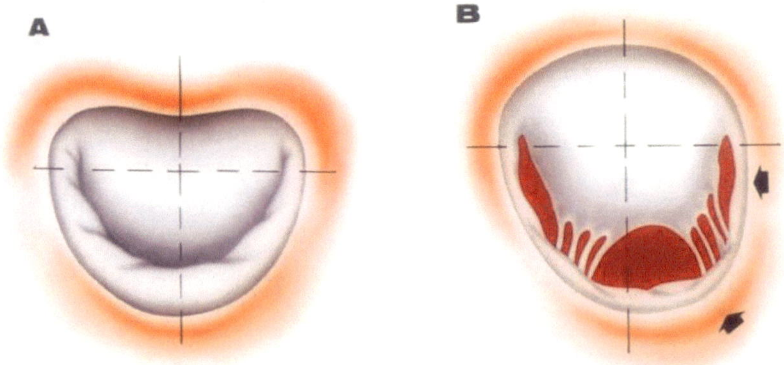

Figure 10. A – Normal mitral valve annulus. B – Posterior dilation of the annulus and to a greater extent next to the postero-medial comissure (arrows).

http://dx.doi.org/10.5772/57114

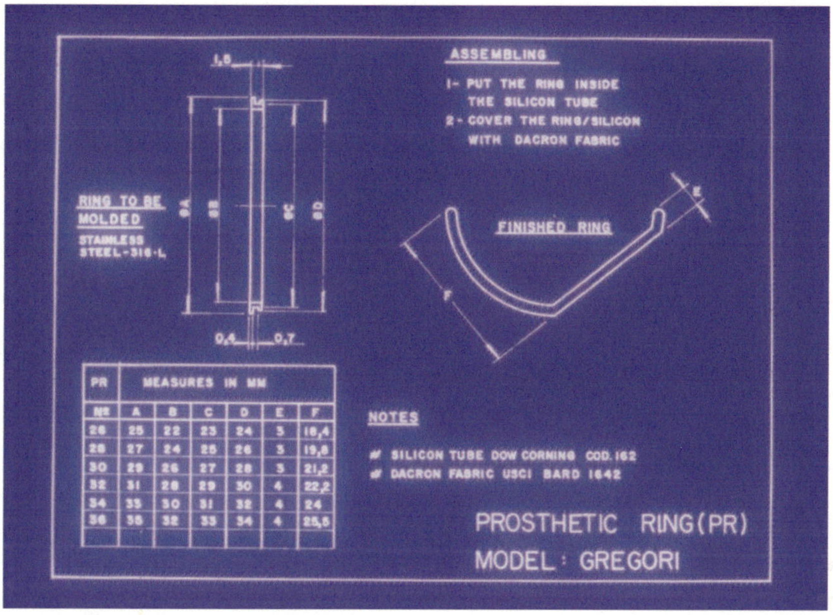

Figure 11. Technical drawing. The assembly of the semi-circular prosthetic ring. Left: measurements of the largest diameter (in millimeters) in A. Right: attention to the rectification on the right that will correct the posterior dilation of the mitral annulus which is greater next to the postero-medial comissure.

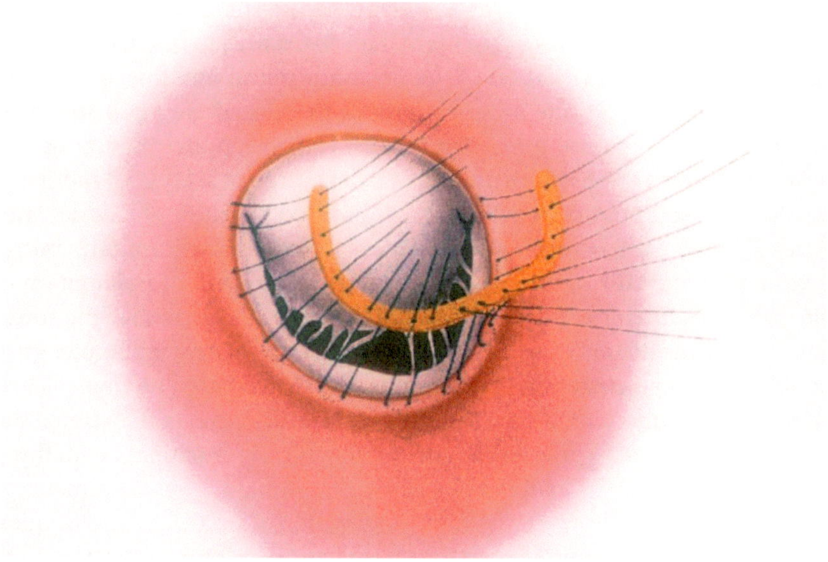

Figure 12. Schematic drawing showing the implantation of the Gregori-Braile Ring prosthesis.

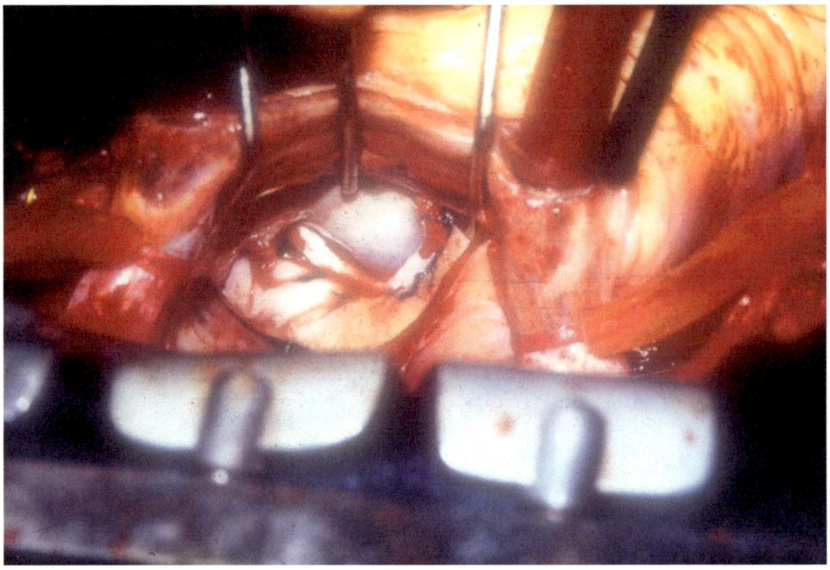

Figure 13. Intraoperative surgical aspect of a mitral annuloplasty by the Gregori-Braile prosthesis ring.

5. Comments

The prosthetic ring presented here was first employed in our Centre in October, 1987 [9]. Since then, this prosthesis has been employed in more than 40 Centres in Brazil and other countries. It was developed to correct the dilation of the posterior mitral annulus, resulting in a semi-circular shape. In our opinion, the anterior part of the closed ring prosthesis is not only dispensable but also inconvenient in some situations. The posterior ring annuloplasty concept has been adopted by many surgeons as described by Hendren et al [10], Salvador et al [11] and Salati et al [12] who used bovine pericardium strips fixed by glutaraldehyde, and by Braile and colleagues [7] who used berets – also made of bovine pericardium. The mitral valvular system, including the mitral ring grows and develops in children. Implantation of an open prosthesis in children with mitral insufficiency allows for normal growth of the anterior leaflet, which corresponds to the distance between the fibrous trigonae. Any millimeter growth in this area may avoid the late manifestation of mitral stenosis, which happens when closed rings are used in small children. Our own comparative studies in adults have demonstrated the presence of a mitral transvalvar pressure gradient of smaller magnitude in patients with this prosthesis when compared to patients who had the closed ring implanted. The adjustment on the right side of the prosthetic ring was introduced for the correction of small leakage, frequently found next to the postero-medial commissure, since this is the portion of the mitral ring with greater dilation. If required, with the Gregori-Braile ring already implanted, intervention on the sub-valvar system is possible with great ease, including the shortening of elongated chordae tendineae and sectioning of retractable chordae.

http://dx.doi.org/10.5772/57114

The results have been consistent both in adults and children. Machado and Gregori (2005) [13] showed the late evaluation of rheumatic children less than 12 years of age submitted to reconstructive mitral valve surgery with implantation of the Gregori-Braile ring. After 188 months, the survival rate was 82% and the annual mortality rate, 0.38%. Thirty-one (72.6%) patients did not require reoperation and the annual rate of patients who required further surgery was 0.51%.

Author details

Francisco Gregori Junior

Cardiac Surgery Division, University of Londrina-Paraná School of Medicine, Brazil

References

[1] Carpentier A, Relland J, Deloche A, Piwinica A, Chauvaud S and Dubost C. Conservative management of the prolapsed mitral valve. Ann Thorac Surg 1978;26:294-302.

[2] Akins CW, Hilgenberg AD, Bukcley MJ, Vlahakes GJ, Torchiana DF, Daggett et al. Mitral valve reconstruction versus replacement for degenerative or ischemic mitral regurgitation. Ann Thorac Surg 1994;58:668-75.

[3] Gregori F Jr, Silva SS, Façanha L, Cordeiro C, Aquino W and Moure O. Preliminary results with a new technique for repairing elongated chordae tendineae of the anterior mitral valve leaflet (Letter). J. Thorac Cardiovasc Surg 1994;107:321-3.

[4] Gregori F Jr, Takeda R, Silva S, Façanha L and Meier MA. A new technique for repair of mitral insufficiency caused by ruptured chordae of the anterior leaflet. J Thorac Cardiovasc Surg 1988;96:765-8.

[5] Gregori F Jr, Cordeiro C, Croti UA, Hayashi SS, Silva SS and Gregori TE. Partial tricuspid valve transfer for repair of mitral insufficiency due to ruptured chordae tendineae. Ann Thorac Surg 1999;68:1686-91

[6] Gregori F Jr, Leal JC and Braile DM. Premolded bovine pericardial chordae for replacement of ruptured or elongated chordae tendineae. Heart Surg Forum. 2010;13:E17-20.

[7] Braile DM, Ardito RV, Pinto GH et al. Plastia mitral. Rev. Bras Cir Cardiovasc 1990;5:86-98

[8] Hueb AC, Jatene FB, Moreira LFP, Pomerantzeff P, Kallás E and Oliveira SA. Ventricular remodeling and mitral valve modifications in dilated cardiomyopathy: New insights from anatomic study. J. Thorac Cardiovasc Surg. 2002;124:1216-24.

[9] Gregori F Jr., Silva SS, Hayashi SS, Aquino W, Cordeiro C, Silva LR.. Mitral valvuloplasty with a new prosthetic ring. Analysis of the first 105 cases. Eur J. Cardiovasc Surg 1994;8:168-72.

[10] Hendren WG, Nemec JJ, Lytle BW, Loop FD, Taylor PC, Stewart RW et al. Mitral valve repair for ischemic mitral insufficiency. Ann Thorac Surg 1991;52:1246-1255

[11] Salvador L, Rocco F and Lus P. The pericardium reinforced suture annuloplasty: Another tool avaiable for mitral annulus repair ? J Cardiovasc Surg 1993;8:79-84

[12] Salati M, Scrofani R, and Santoli C. Posterior pericardial annuloplasty: a physiological correction ?. Eur J Cardiothorac Surg 1991;5:226-9.

[13] Machado VH and Gregori F Jr. Late heart evaluation of children with rheumatic mitral regurgitation submitted to reconstructive surgery with implantation of Gregori's Ring. (in Portuguese) Arq Bras Cardiol. 2005;85:403-11.

Chapter 5

Coronary Artery Bypass Grafting Without Cardiopulmonary Bypass and Without Aortic Manipulation

José Glauco Lobo Filho,
Heraldo Guedis Lobo Filho and
Eduardo Rebouças Carvalho

Additional information is available at the end of the chapter

http://dx.doi.org/10.5772/57115

1. Introduction

The methods for coronary artery bypass grafting (CABG) have evolved rapidly in recent years. Procedures such as the CABG without cardiopulmonary bypass (CPB), non-handling of the ascending aorta (AA) and the search for better grafts are strategies that aim at reducing the morbidity and mortality in the immediate postoperative period, the reduction of hospital stay and the increase in expectation and quality of life of patients on long-term [1].

It is known that changes, especially at the cellular level, resulting from the blood flow by non-endothelial surfaces in cardiopulmonary bypass (CPB), trigger the systemic inflammatory response syndrome [2, 3]. The use of CPB, and inflammatory disorders, can cause coagulation disorders with procoagulant effects and may cause early obstruction of the grafts [4], cerebral embolic events with irreversible neurological damage [5-8], and susceptibility to infectious processes due to immune depression in postoperative period [9].

The handling of AA is intrinsically related to the occurrence of cerebrovascular accident (stroke), especially in elderly patients, either at the time of cannulation, clamping and un-clamping of the aorta to the installation and maintenance of the CPB circuit, to carry out the proximal anastomosis of vascular grafts [10-12]. Some studies show that the handling of AA is not the most important factor in reducing neurological complications [13, 14].

Another important factor for the improvement of CABG in the long term is the selection of the grafts and the configuration thereof. It should be taken into account the specific anatomical and clinical conditions of each patient and the surgical team's experience in obtaining, preparation and anastomosis of the grafts.

The use of composite graft setting in "Y", the left internal thoracic artery (LITA) with arterial segments or segments of great saphenous vein (GSV) to revascularize both the left coronary system (LCS) as the right is a technique widely described in literature, especially in patients at high risk of stroke [15]. This procedure can be performed without CPB and without manipulation of the AA, being the LITA the main source of blood supply to more than one coronary artery. The LITA, in turn can also be used sequentially to the grafting of two or three arteries of the left anterior descending artery (AD), being able to provide adequate blood supply for the entire LCS, both at rest and stress [16].

Although the use of the GSV as aortocoronary graft is related to higher incidence of obstructions than arterial grafts, especially the LITA, in short, medium and long-term disease called aorto-coronary vein graft [17], it seems likely that the use valveless GSV segments in combination with the LITA may modify these results [18, 19]. In our department we use routinely a composite graft of LIMA and valveless GSV, in "Y" for the revascularization of arteries of the LCS.

2. Surgical technique for CABG without CPB and without AA manipulation using composite graft

After electrocardiographic monitoring of central venous pressure and mean arterial pressure, the patient is anesthetized. Proceeding to the opening of the chest (sternotomy or left thoracotomy), exposing finally the heart, the pericardium by setting the drapes. The LITA is completely dissected from its origin until the seventh intercostal space, making up ligation of all branches possible with a metal clip. Obtaining the saphenous vein graft is done preferentially by endoscopic dissection [20]. The procedure is anticoagulation by intravenous administration of sodium heparin at doses of 1.0 mg / kg body weight, with accurate control of the activated clotting time, which must be greater than 200 seconds [21]. We emphasize that both the perfusionist as all the equipment for immediate installation of the CPB circuit is available to the surgical team.

Being the grafts properly prepared, the coronary arteries to be grafted are dissected. The interruption of blood flow to regions of the coronary arteries, where anastomosis shall be made is performed by passing a 5-0 polypropylene line, in eight, with tourniquets proximal and distal to the anastomosis site. Among the coronary and tourniquets, in order to protect the coronary arterial bed, it is interposed a small segment (1.0 cm) of silicone tubes (Figure 1). The intracoronary perfusates are only used in special situations.

The coronary artery is incised longitudinally, and anastomosis performed with the aid of a tissue stabilizer (Figure 1), using a single polypropylene line 7-0 or 8-0 in cases of venous grafts and 8-0 in the case of arterial grafts. Invariably, the LITA is anastomosed to the AD, and one segment GSV, originating from the side of the LITA, revascularizes a second branch of the LCS

http://dx.doi.org/10.5772/57115

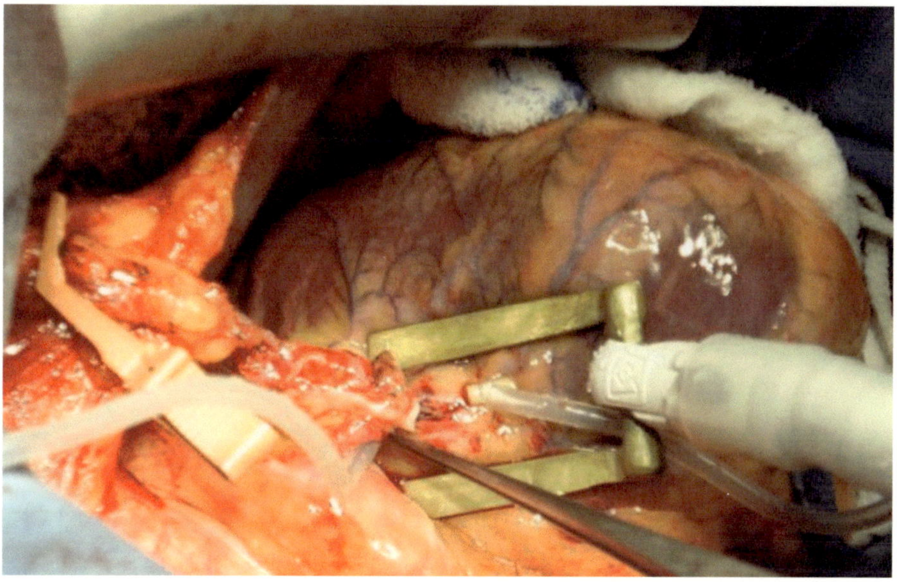

Figure 1. Protection of the coronary arterial bed with a small silicone tube segment number 10 on the occasion of the coronary tourniquet. Device for stabilizing tissue in the anastomosis.

(Figures 2 and 3). For revascularization of the posterior arteries, we used the Lima Point, which facilitates the rotation of the mediastinum to the right [22].

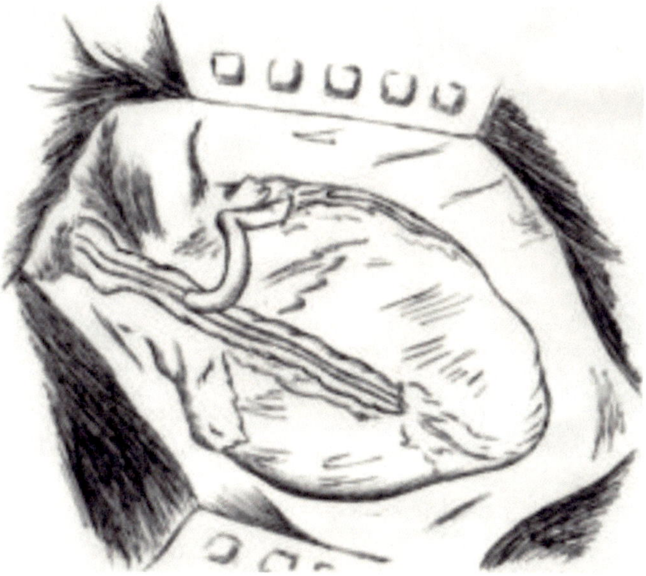

Figure 2. Schematic of a composite graft of LITA with GSV revascularizing the AD and a marginal circumflex artery, respectively

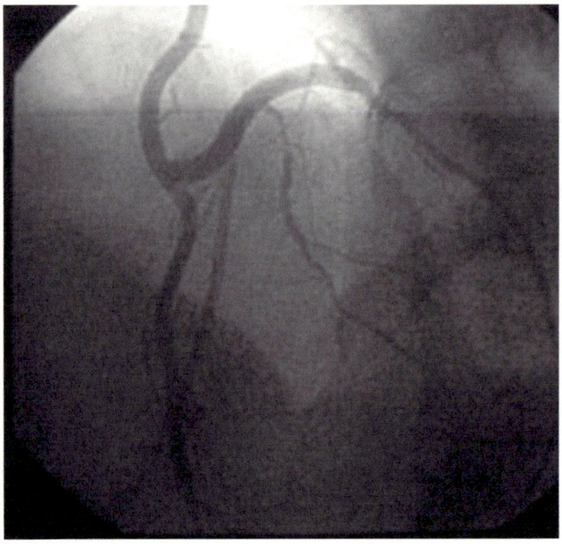

Figure 3. Angiographic study of a composite graft of LITA revascularizing AD and one segment GSV originated from a LITA revascularizing the circumflex marginal artery. Left anterior oblique cranial flow.

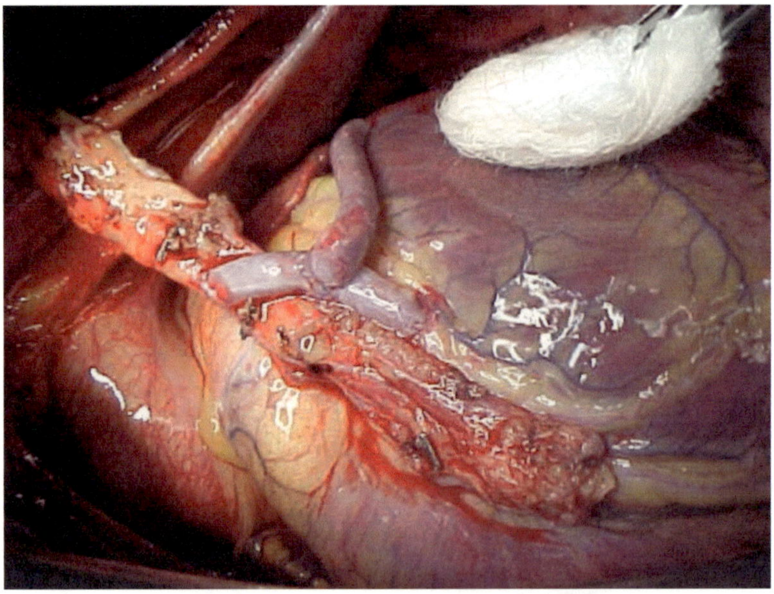

Figure 4. Schematic of a composite graft of LITA revascularizing AD and a GSV segment derived from the LITA revascularizing the 1st Diagonal and a second segment originating from GSV revascularizing a diagonal of the circumflex marginal artery.

When other branches need to be revascularized, a second vein segment stems from the anterior side of the vein segment (Figures 4 and 5). The venous segment can also be anastomosed sequentially. The evaluation of the flow of the grafts after preparing the same, using flowmetry instruments is of paramount importance, being routinely performed in various facilities.

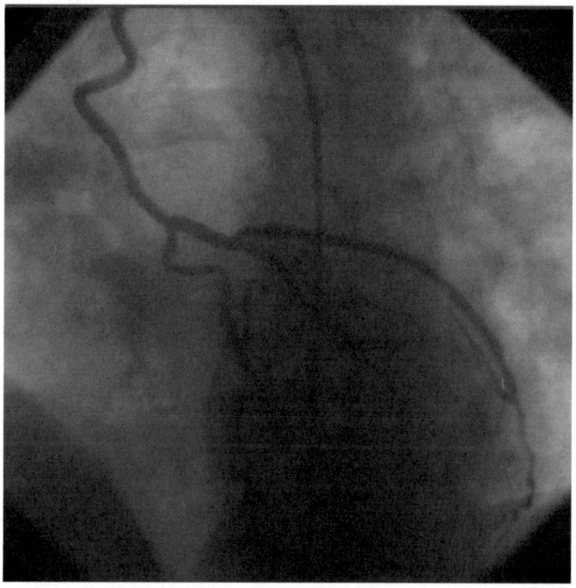

Figure 5. Angiography of a composite graft of LITA revascularizing AD and a GSV segment derived from the LITA revascularizing the 1st Diagonal and a second segment originating from the GSV revascularizing a diagonal of the circumflex marginal artery. Examination 11 years after surgery.

3. Final considerations

In our department, since the mid-1990s, is routinely performed Off Pump Coronary artery Bypass (OPCAB) surgery in 92% of patients with stable coronary artery disease. This associated with the frequent use of LITA grafts composed of GSV and arteries for revascularization of the LCS, with excellent results in terms of morbidity and Doppler or angiographic evaluation of grafts in the short, medium and long term [23-25].

In the preoperative approach of patients we considered critically important the nutritional and medicinal aspects. The reduction of sodium intake and calorie foods, weight loss, regarding the increase of food of real nutrition and immunomodulator value are important. The administration of statins, acetylsalicylic acid (ASA), beta-blockers is maintained until the day before surgery, because they are related to the reduction of inflammatory response, lower incidence of early thrombosis of grafts and prevention of atrial fibrillation in the post- surgery. Glycemic control is done strictly to prevent infectious complications [26].

Regarding the preoperative examinations all patients underwent echocardiography, Doppler study by the carotid and vertebral arteries and the venous system of lower limbs and abdominal ultrasound evaluation, for abdominal aortic aneurysm screening.

Regarding the operative aspects, we think the two biggest factors that increase morbidity and mortality in CABG surgery is the use of CPB and the handling of AA. The CPB, as has been explained, is related to inflammatory changes that may result in exacerbated systemic inflammatory response syndrome affecting multiple organic. Studies clearly demonstrate the association of CPB with brain [27], lung [28], kidney [29] and gastrointestinal [30] damage.

The CPB is still associated with higher levels of bleeding during and after surgery and therefore with greater administration of blood products [31]. The use of these agents in turn, its associated, in addition to the known complications of immunologic and infectious nature, to the lower long-term survival [32]. Another important fact is that in OPCAB the dose of heparin required for anticoagulation is small enough to achieve an activated clotting time greater than 200 seconds, thus the dose of protamine administered at the end of the procedure will be lower, because this drug is related to a series of negative effects on the hemodynamic and inflammatory aspect [33].

The handling of AA, as well discussed, is intrinsically linked to embolic events when there is atheromatous disease of the ascending aorta. However, beyond this fact, the partial or total clamping of the aorta can cause aortic dissection [34].

In an era when one seeks a broader use of arterial grafts one might ask why the routine use of GSV associated with LITA. First one must take into account the morbidity associated with obtaining the grafts. Mediastinitis is a terrible complication associated with increased mortality, with devastating consequences to the physical and psychological integrity of the patient as well as repercussions in terms of financial cost on the public or private health system [35]. The use of two LITAs doubles the risk of internal thoracic mediastinitis compared to the use of a single LITA [36] and can increase up to fourteen times the risk of this complication associated with diabetes mellitus [37].

Regarding the use of the radial artery it is described that its dissection causes neurological complications in about 30 percent of patients [38]. The radial artery is an artery muscle spasm and susceptible to atrophy, especially when used to revascularize the coronary arteries without severe stenosis [39, 40]. It is noteworthy that the angiographic results of radial artery grafts are not superior to that of GSV grafts [41]. Obtaining gastroepiploic artery, in turn, brings the disadvantage of opening of the peritoneal cavity, and similarly to the radial artery, it is prone to spasm and thus it is only used for the revascularization of severe stenosed arteries [42].

Obtaining the GSV causes minimal morbidity, especially when done in an endoscopic manner. It is a long graft, easy to handle and has no tendency to spasm. We consider of utmost importance the venous Doppler study of lower limb in order to ascertain the GSV along its entire length, the presence of valves and varicosities, and mark its location to better perform the incisions for the dissection, with less tissue trauma and preservation of cosmetic and finally the possibility of the preoperative preparation of another option, in those patients in which GSV is not considered appropriate [43].

The obstruction of the GSV grafts occurs mainly by the action of three factors, which are thrombosis, intimal hyperplasia and atherosclerosis [4, 44]. We think that the saphenous vein, the way we use it, can have a better behavior than those currently described, for the following reasons:

1. The CABG procedure performed without CPB and, especially in the presence of AAS, has a lower prothrombotic nature, which should be associated with lower rates of occlusion of graft thrombosis [45].

2. The SV segments that we use are small and without valves, reducing the resistance to blood flow and eliminating sites (valves) that favor the development of stenosis [4, 18, 46];

3. Lower blood pressure and circulatory stress imposed on segments of the saphenous vein from the LITA, compared to those originating from the aorta, might cause less damage to the intimate, less development of intimal hyperplasia and atherosclerosis [47, 48];

4. As the endothelium of the LITA is a major producer of nitric oxide, we believe that the SV graft, originating from this artery, may receive part of this hormone, thereby decreasing the incidence of atherosclerotic disease [44, 49];

5. hemodynamically the presence of the valve in the GSV segment can primarily cause entrapment of blood between the coronary anastomosis and the valve due to the phenomenon of flow, natural in the blood circulatory system, with increasing pressure during diastole with consequent stagnation of flow in venous segment; secondarily this flow stagnation limits the infusion, in order to generate a vicious cycle, leading to obstruction of the graft. This mechanism becomes responsible for 20% of cases of graft failure following a year [18, 46].

In order to reduce the heart rate and decrease the energy consumption of the cardiomyocyte during anastomoses, especially of the LITA to the AD, we administered esmolol, beta-blocker of quick action, which has duration of action of about nine minutes. We believe that the use of this drug to integrates the concept of myocardial protection in CABG surgery without CPB [50].

The increasing popularity of off-pump CABG surgery has brought concern, especially in groups that start in the use of this technique, with the quality of anastomoses. Methods for verification of graft patency in the intraoperative period are not commonly performed, and most cardiovascular surgeons rely on electrocardiographic criteria, and hemodynamic enzyme to make a diagnosis of early occlusion of grafts. The use of Transit-time flowmetry has been adopted in many centers for CABG surgery with or without CPB [51].

In cases of elective surgery, epidural anesthesia with opioids and local anesthetic is routinely performed. This procedure has a number of benefits beyond the appropriate component of postoperative analgesia, such as increasing the diameter of epicardial arteries, improves flow through collateral circulation, reduction of myocardial oxygen demand, decreased arrhythmias, lower rates of sternum infection and modulation of inflammatory activity [52, 53].

For the future we aim to allow our patients the benefits of revascularization by left minithoracotomy with the aid of thoracoscopy [54] for cases of revascularization of arteries of the LCS with or without percutaneous treatment of lesions of the right coronary artery or other vessels [55]. We are still attentive to the evolution of epicardial ablation treatment for atrial fibrillation

[56], as well as the development of efficient devices to exclude the left atrial appendage, focus formation and embolization of 60-91%% of thrombi causing embolic ischemic stroke in validity of this tachyarrhythmia [57].

Finally, we believe that surgical revascularization of the LCS can be systematically performed without CPB and without manipulation of the AA, in order to reduce the systemic inflammatory response, blood transfusion, and mortality, particularly related to neurological complications. Furthermore, the use of a valveless GSV grafts associated with LITA for coronary artery bypass grafting of the LCS simplifies the technique of anastomosis "Y", making it more physiological and, it may also be associated with a higher rate of graft patency in the long term.

Author details

José Glauco Lobo Filho, Heraldo Guedis Lobo Filho and Eduardo Rebouças Carvalho

Hospital Sao Raimundo, Fortaleza, Ceará CE, Brazil

References

[1] Hillis LD, Smith PK, Anderson JL, Bittl JA, Bridges CR, Byrne JG, et al. 2011 ACCF/AHA Guideline for Coronary Artery Bypass Graft Surgery. A report of the American College of Cardiology Foundation/American Heart Association Task Force on Practice Guidelines. Developed in collaboration with the American Association for Thoracic Surgery, Society of Cardiovascular Anesthesiologists, and Society of Thoracic Surgeons. Journal of the American College of Cardiology. 2011;58[24):e123-210. Epub 2011/11/11.

[2] Kirklin JK, Westaby S, Blackstone EH, Kirklin JW, Chenoweth DE, Pacifico AD. Complement and the damaging effects of cardiopulmonary bypass. The Journal of thoracic and cardiovascular surgery. 1983;86[6):845-57. Epub 1983/12/01.

[3] Ascione R, Lloyd CT, Underwood MJ, Lotto AA, Pitsis AA, Angelini GD. Inflammatory response after coronary revascularization with or without cardiopulmonary bypass. The Annals of thoracic surgery. 2000;69[4):1198-204. Epub 2000/05/09.

[4] Motwani JG, Topol EJ. Aortocoronary saphenous vein graft disease: pathogenesis, predisposition, and prevention. Circulation. 1998;97[9):916-31. Epub 1998/04/01.

[5] Blauth CI, Arnold JV, Schulenberg WE, McCartney AC, Taylor KM. Cerebral microembolism during cardiopulmonary bypass. Retinal microvascular studies in vivo with fluorescein angiography. The Journal of thoracic and cardiovascular surgery. 1988;95[4):668-76. Epub 1988/04/01.

[6] Harringer W. Capture of particulate emboli during cardiac procedures in which aortic cross-clamp is used. International Council of Emboli Management Study Group. The Annals of thoracic surgery. 2000;70[3]:1119-23. Epub 2000/10/04.

[7] Newman MF, Kirchner JL, Phillips-Bute B, Gaver V, Grocott H, Jones RH, et al. Longitudinal assessment of neurocognitive function after coronary-artery bypass surgery. The New England journal of medicine. 2001;344[6]:395-402. Epub 2001/02/15.

[8] Groom RC, Quinn RD, Lennon P, Welch J, Kramer RS, Ross CS, et al. Microemboli from cardiopulmonary bypass are associated with a serum marker of brain injury. The Journal of extra-corporeal technology. 2010;42[1]:40-4. Epub 2010/05/05.

[9] Akbas H, Erdal AC, Demiralp E, Alp M. Effects of coronary artery bypass grafting on cellular immunity with or without cardiopulmonary bypass: changes in lymphocytes subsets. Cardiovascular surgery (London, England). 2002;10[6]:586-9. Epub 2002/11/28.

[10] Barbut D, Hinton RB, Szatrowski TP, Hartman GS, Bruefach M, Williams-Russo P, et al. Cerebral emboli detected during bypass surgery are associated with clamp removal. Stroke; a journal of cerebral circulation. 1994;25[12]:2398-402. Epub 1994/12/01.

[11] Dietl CA, Madigan NP, Laubach CA, Chapman JH, Bering JP, Holcomb PH, et al. Myocardial revascularization using the "no-touch" technique, with mild systemic hypothermia, in patients with a calcified ascending aorta. The Journal of cardiovascular surgery. 1995;36[1]:39-44. Epub 1995/02/01.

[12] Trehan N, Mishra M, Kasliwal RR, Mishra A. Surgical strategies in patients at high risk for stroke undergoing coronary artery bypass grafting. The Annals of thoracic surgery. 2000;70[3]:1037-45. Epub 2000/10/04.

[13] Lev-Ran O, Loberman D, Matsa M, Pevni D, Nesher N, Mohr R, et al. Reduced strokes in the elderly: the benefits of untouched aorta off-pump coronary surgery. The Annals of thoracic surgery. 2004;77[1]:102-7. Epub 2004/01/17.

[14] Misfeld M, Potger K, Ross DE, McMillan D, Brady PW, Marshman D, et al. "Anaortic" off-pump coronary artery bypass grafting significantly reduces neurological complications compared to off-pump and conventional on-pump surgery with aortic manipulation. The Thoracic and cardiovascular surgeon. 2010;58[7]:408-14. Epub 2010/10/06.

[15] Wendler O, Hennen B, Markwirth T, Konig J, Tscholl D, Huang Q, et al. T grafts with the right internal thoracic artery to left internal thoracic artery versus the left internal thoracic artery and radial artery: flow dynamics in the internal thoracic artery main stem. The Journal of thoracic and cardiovascular surgery. 1999;118[5]:841-8. Epub 1999/10/27.

[16] Lobo Filho JG, Leitão MCdA, Lobo Filho HG, Silva AAd, Machado JJA, Forte AJdV, et al. Revascularização miocárdica com enxerto composto de artéria torácica interna

esquerda em Y: análise de fluxo sangüíneo. Revista Brasileira de Cirurgia Cardiovascular. 2004;19:1-8.

[17] Sabik JF, 3rd, Lytle BW, Blackstone EH, Houghtaling PL, Cosgrove DM. Comparison of saphenous vein and internal thoracic artery graft patency by coronary system. The Annals of thoracic surgery. 2005;79[2):544-51; discussion -51. Epub 2005/02/01.

[18] Lajos TZ, Robicsek F, Thubrikar M, Urschel H. Improving patency of coronary conduits "valveless" veins and/or arterial grafts. Journal of cardiac surgery. 2007;22[2): 170-7. Epub 2007/03/07.

[19] Hwang HY, Kim JS, Kim KB. Angiographic equivalency of off-pump saphenous vein and arterial composite grafts at one year. The Annals of thoracic surgery. 2010;90[2): 516-21. Epub 2010/07/30.

[20] Black EA, Campbell RK, Channon KM, Ratnatunga C, Pillai R. Minimally invasive vein harvesting significantly reduces pain and wound morbidity. European journal of cardio-thoracic surgery : official journal of the European Association for Cardio-thoracic Surgery. 2002;22[3):381-6. Epub 2002/09/03.

[21] Lobo Filho JG, Leitão MC, Lobo RAM, Lima Júnior JMd, Ribeiro JPA, Cavalcante F, et al. Padronização da dose de heparina sódica utilizada na cirurgia de revascularização do miocárdio sem circulação extracorpórea. Revista Brasileira de Cirurgia Cardiovascular. 2005;20:279-85.

[22] Lima RC. Padronização técnica de revascularização miocárdica da artéria circunflexa e seus ramos sem circulação extracorpórea. São Paulo. Tese [Doutorado]. Escola Paulista de Medicina da USP; 1999.

[23] Lobo Filho JG, Dantas MCBR, Rolim JGV, Rocha JA, Oliveira FM, Ciarline C, et al. Cirurgia de revascularização completa do miocárdio sem circulação extracorpórea: uma realidade. Rev Bras Cir Cardiovasc. 1997;12:7.

[24] Lobo Filho JG, Leitao MC, Lobo Filho HG, Soares JPH, Magalhães GA, Leao Filho CSC, et al. Cirurgia de revascularização coronariana esquerda sem CEC e sem manuseio da aorta em pacientes acima de 75 anos: análise das mortalidades imediata e a médio prazo e das complicações neurológicas no pós-operatório imediato. Rev Bras Cir Cardiovasc. 2002;17:6.

[25] Lobo Filho JG, Leitao MC, Forte AJ, Filho HG, Silva AA, Bastos ES, et al. Flow analysis of left internal thoracic artery in myocardial revascularization surgery using y graft. Texas Heart Institute journal / from the Texas Heart Institute of St Luke's Episcopal Hospital, Texas Children's Hospital. 2006;33[4):430-6. Epub 2007/01/12.

[26] Ingels C, Debaveye Y, Milants I, Buelens E, Peeraer A, Devriendt Y, et al. Strict blood glucose control with insulin during intensive care after cardiac surgery: impact on 4-years survival, dependency on medical care, and quality-of-life. European heart journal. 2006;27[22):2716-24. Epub 2006/04/13.

[27] Taylor KM. Brain damage during cardiopulmonary bypass. The Annals of thoracic surgery. 1998;65[4 Suppl):S20-6; discussion S7-8. Epub 1998/05/01.

[28] Apostolakis EE, Koletsis EN, Baikoussis NG, Siminelakis SN, Papadopoulos GS. Strategies to prevent intraoperative lung injury during cardiopulmonary bypass. Journal of cardiothoracic surgery. 2010;5:1. Epub 2010/01/13.

[29] Abu-Omar Y, Ratnatunga C. Cardiopulmonary bypass and renal injury. Perfusion. 2006;21[4):209-13. Epub 2006/08/31.

[30] Sinclair DG, Haslam PL, Quinlan GJ, Pepper JR, Evans TW. The effect of cardiopulmonary bypass on intestinal and pulmonary endothelial permeability. Chest. 1995;108[3):718-24. Epub 1995/09/01.

[31] Coakley M, Hall JE, Evans C, Duff E, Billing V, Yang L, et al. Assessment of thrombin generation measured before and after cardiopulmonary bypass surgery and its association with postoperative bleeding. Journal of thrombosis and haemostasis : JTH. 2011;9[2):282-92. Epub 2010/11/26.

[32] Engoren MC, Habib RH, Zacharias A, Schwann TA, Riordan CJ, Durham SJ. Effect of blood transfusion on long-term survival after cardiac operation. The Annals of thoracic surgery. 2002;74[4):1180-6. Epub 2002/10/29.

[33] Viaro F, Dalio MB, Evora PR. Catastrophic cardiovascular adverse reactions to protamine are nitric oxide/cyclic guanosine monophosphate dependent and endothelium mediated: should methylene blue be the treatment of choice? Chest. 2002;122[3): 1061-6. Epub 2002/09/13.

[34] Litchford B, Okies JE, Sugimura S, Starr A. Acute aortic dissection from cross-clamp injury. The Journal of thoracic and cardiovascular surgery. 1976;72[5):709-13. Epub 1976/11/01.

[35] Nina VJdS, Assef MAS, Rodrigues RR, Mendes VGG, Lages JS, Amorim ÂMM, et al. Reconstrução da parede torácica com suporte metálico externo: técnica alternativa na mediastinite pós-esternotomia. Revista Brasileira de Cirurgia Cardiovascular. 2008;23:507-11.

[36] Grossi EA, Esposito R, Harris LJ, Crooke GA, Galloway AC, Colvin SB, et al. Sternal wound infections and use of internal mammary artery grafts. The Journal of thoracic and cardiovascular surgery. 1991;102[3):342-6; discussion 6-7. Epub 1991/09/01.

[37] Borger MA, Rao V, Weisel RD, Ivanov J, Cohen G, Scully HE, et al. Deep sternal wound infection: risk factors and outcomes. The Annals of thoracic surgery. 1998;65[4):1050-6. Epub 1998/05/16.

[38] Denton TA, Trento L, Cohen M, Kass RM, Blanche C, Raissi S, et al. Radial artery harvesting for coronary bypass operations: neurologic complications and their potential mechanisms. The Journal of thoracic and cardiovascular surgery. 2001;121[5):951-6. Epub 2001/04/28.

[39] Maniar HS, Sundt TM, Barner HB, Prasad SM, Peterson L, Absi T, et al. Effect of target stenosis and location on radial artery graft patency. The Journal of thoracic and cardiovascular surgery. 2002;123[1):45-52. Epub 2002/01/10.

[40] Moran SV, Baeza R, Guarda E, Zalaquett R, Irarrazaval MJ, Marchant E, et al. Predictors of radial artery patency for coronary bypass operations. The Annals of thoracic surgery. 2001;72[5):1552-6. Epub 2001/11/28.

[41] Locali RF, Buffolo E, Catani R. Artéria radial versus veia safena para revascularização do miocárdio: metanálise (não houve diferença estatisticamente significante). Revista Brasileira de Cirurgia Cardiovascular. 2006;21:255-61.

[42] Glineur D, D'Hoore W, El Khoury G, Sondji S, Kalscheuer G, Funken JC, et al. Angiographic predictors of 6-month patency of bypass grafts implanted to the right coronary artery a prospective randomized comparison of gastroepiploic artery and saphenous vein grafts. Journal of the American College of Cardiology. 2008;51[2): 120-5. Epub 2008/01/15.

[43] BARROS FS, PONTES SM, LIMA ML, HENRIQUE JS, ROLDI ML, REIS F, et al. Mapeamento da safena interna com ecocolor Doppler no pré-operatório de cirurgia de revascularização miocárdica. Revista Brasileira de Cirurgia Cardiovascular. 1999;14:303-7.

[44] Nwasokwa ON. Coronary artery bypass graft disease. Annals of internal medicine. 1995;123[7):528-45. Epub 1995/10/01.

[45] Paparella D, Galeone A, Venneri MT, Coviello M, Scrascia G, Marraudino N, et al. Activation of the coagulation system during coronary artery bypass grafting: comparison between on-pump and off-pump techniques. The Journal of thoracic and cardiovascular surgery. 2006;131[2):290-7. Epub 2006/01/26.

[46] Lajos TZ, Graham SP, Guntupalli M, Raza ST, Hasnain S. Comparison of long-term patency of "horseshoe" saphenous vein grafts with and without valves. European journal of cardio-thoracic surgery : official journal of the European Association for Cardio-thoracic Surgery. 1996;10[10):846-51. Epub 1996/01/01.

[47] Nguyen HC, Grossi EA, LeBoutillier M, 3rd, Steinberg BM, Rifkin DB, Baumann FG, et al. Mammary artery versus saphenous vein grafts: assessment of basic fibroblast growth factor receptors. The Annals of thoracic surgery. 1994;58[2):308-10; discussion 10-1. Epub 1994/08/01.

[48] Calafiore AM, Vitolla G, Iaco AL, Fino C, Di Giammarco G, Marchesani F, et al. Bilateral internal mammary artery grafting: midterm results of pedicled versus skeletonized conduits. The Annals of thoracic surgery. 1999;67[6):1637-42. Epub 1999/07/03.

[49] Shuhaiber JH, Evans AN, Massad MG, Geha AS. Mechanisms and future directions for prevention of vein graft failure in coronary bypass surgery. European journal of

cardio-thoracic surgery : official journal of the European Association for Cardio-thoracic Surgery. 2002;22[3):387-96. Epub 2002/09/03.

[50] Chassot PG, van der Linden P, Zaugg M, Mueller XM, Spahn DR. Off-pump coronary artery bypass surgery: physiology and anaesthetic management. British journal of anaesthesia. 2004;92[3):400-13. Epub 2004/02/19.

[51] D'Ancona G, Karamanoukian HL, Ricci M, Schmid S, Bergsland J, Salerno TA. Graft revision after transit time flow measurement in off-pump coronary artery bypass grafting. European journal of cardio-thoracic surgery : official journal of the European Association for Cardio-thoracic Surgery. 2000;17[3):287-93. Epub 2000/04/12.

[52] Kirno K, Friberg P, Grzegorczyk A, Milocco I, Ricksten SE, Lundin S. Thoracic epidural anesthesia during coronary artery bypass surgery: effects on cardiac sympathetic activity, myocardial blood flow and metabolism, and central hemodynamics. Anesthesia and analgesia. 1994;79[6):1075-81. Epub 1994/12/01.

[53] Scott NB, Turfrey DJ, Ray DA, Nzewi O, Sutcliffe NP, Lal AB, et al. A prospective randomized study of the potential benefits of thoracic epidural anesthesia and analgesia in patients undergoing coronary artery bypass grafting. Anesthesia and analgesia. 2001;93[3):528-35. Epub 2001/08/29.

[54] Lima LE, Nataf P, Lima AE, Franceschini IA, Gomes C, Paniagua P, et al. Técnica de revascularização miocárdica com uso de toracoscopia. Revista Brasileira de Cirurgia Cardiovascular. 1996;11:232-7.

[55] DeRose JJ. Current state of integrated "hybrid" coronary revascularization. Seminars in thoracic and cardiovascular surgery. 2009;21[3):229-36. Epub 2009/11/28.

[56] Ninet J, Roques X, Seitelberger R, Deville C, Pomar JL, Robin J, et al. Surgical ablation of atrial fibrillation with off-pump, epicardial, high-intensity focused ultrasound: results of a multicenter trial. The Journal of thoracic and cardiovascular surgery. 2005;130[3):803-9. Epub 2005/09/13.

[57] Gillinov AM. Advances in surgical treatment of atrial fibrillation. Stroke; a journal of cerebral circulation. 2007;38[2 Suppl):618-23. Epub 2007/01/31.

Chapter 6

Use of Inhaled Nitric Oxide in Cardiac Surgery: What is Going on?

Alfredo José Rodrigues, Patricia Martinez Evora and
Paulo Roberto Barbosa Evora

Additional information is available at the end of the chapter

http://dx.doi.org/10.5772/57109

1. Introduction

In the eighties, the mere finding that acetylcholine only acts as a vasodilator in the presence of the endothelium, established its pivotal role in the physiopathology of cardiovascular diseases. Therefore, the existence of an endothelium-derived relaxing factor [1], which in 1982 was named "endothelium-derived relaxing factor" (EDRF) [2], was postulated. Using endothelial cell culture it was found that endothelium-dependent relaxation was associated with an increase of cyclic GMP (cGMP) in vascular smooth muscle, which could be inhibited by methylene blue (soluble guanylate cyclase) and hemoglobin (EDRF "scavenger").[3] With the accumulation of evidence that EDRF had characteristics similar to nitrovasodilators, Furchgott and Ignarro, [4,5] independently, proposed that EDRF was nitric oxide (NO). The research then was directed in order to determine how the endothelium itself produces the radical and presents the idea of Palmer and Moncada [6,7] postulating that L-arginine is the source of NO under the action of enzyme nitric oxide synthase (NOS).

The hypothesis that inhaled NO could cause selective vasodilatation was based on experimental models of pulmonary hypertension. [8-11] These studies have shown that concentrations of 5 to 80 ppm produced rapid and reversible pulmonary vasodilatation without systemic side effects or adverse reactions. In the lung, as elsewhere in the body, the NO formed from L-arginine in a reaction catalyzed by NO synthase induces vasodilatation through a cGMP-dependent pathway. Nitric oxide can be used by inhalation, acting selectively on those blood vessels near the alveoli. As it undergoes rapid inactivation by hemoglobin, inhaled NO can perform a selective pulmonary vasodilatation were occurring pulmonary vasoconstriction without causing systemic vasodilatation.

The existence of an NO-dependent vascular tone has led to the demonstration that its removal, resulting in "up-regulation" of receptors linked to the NO release pathway, results in increased sensitivity to vasodilators that act through this pathway. The pulmonary vascular bed typically has a low flow resistance. Hypertension in this area may be due to postcapillary blockage or increased flow for this system. When it persists for a long time, this situation leads to secondary changes in these vessels, where proliferation of the muscular layer, fibrosis and obliteration of light are observed. This framework, now irreversible, is associated with high morbidity and mortality. Surgical repair of heart disease should be attempted while the pulmonary vascular system is still responsive. A preoperative evaluation of responsiveness may be possible with NO inhalation. The use of systemic vasodilators can cause unwanted complications such as hypotension, aggravation of a right-left shunt and an underestimation of the real potential of the vasodilator action over the pulmonary bed. Similarly, inhalation of NO may be useful in handling situations of complex control, such as the pulmonary vasospasm observed in the postoperative period of some cardiac surgeries, reducing the right ventricle overload and improving oxygenation.

Because of the rapid inactivation by hemoglobin, and its short half-life, inhaled NO should allow selective pulmonary vasodilatation when there is a vasoconstriction secondary to endothelial dysfunction, or as a result of a potent vasoconstrictive effect.[12-14]

Nitric oxide should provide better oxygenation in the existence of balanced perfusion and ventilation, therefore, having advantages over venous administered vasodilators, which can cause hypotension and increased intrapulmonary "shunt".

The efficacy of inhaled NO in patients with endothelium NO release impairment raises the question if the endogenously release is responsible for increasing the pulmonary vascular tone.[13] NO would be released continuously under the baseline conditions, and the inhibition of this basal release could lead to an increased vascular resistance.[15] The infusion of human lungs with methylene blue alone, an inhibitor of NO-mediated vasorelaxation, leads to an increase in the pulmonary vascular resistance.[16] Thus, pulmonary endothelial damage should be considered when pulmonary vasoconstriction is a consequence of the disease (ARDS - Adult Respiratory Distress Syndrome) or a reversible side effect of treatment (cardiopulmonary "bypass").

Inhaled NO action, different from the NO intravenous action, is limited to veins and arteries of small resistance, and is unable to dilate large capacitance vessels.[17] In lungs, inhaled NO acts primarily on the arterial vessels, but can, during high venous vasoconstriction, also act in the postcapillary bed. In adults with acute lung disease, NO has a vasodilator effect mainly in the venous vascularity.[18] This increased responsiveness appears in pediatric patients with pulmonary venous hypertension, in which the NO should lead to vasodilatation with a combination of pre and post capillary vessels.

The development of right ventricular failure secondary to pulmonary arterial hypertension is a serious postoperative complication of cardiac surgery in children and adults. The selective pulmonary vasodilatation produced by inhaled NO is a therapeutic option that, in certain situations, can be crucial in managing this condition. NO binds to hemoglobin, resulting in its systemic inactivation, resulting in the preservation of coronary and systemic blood pressures (Figure 1).

http://dx.doi.org/10.5772/57109

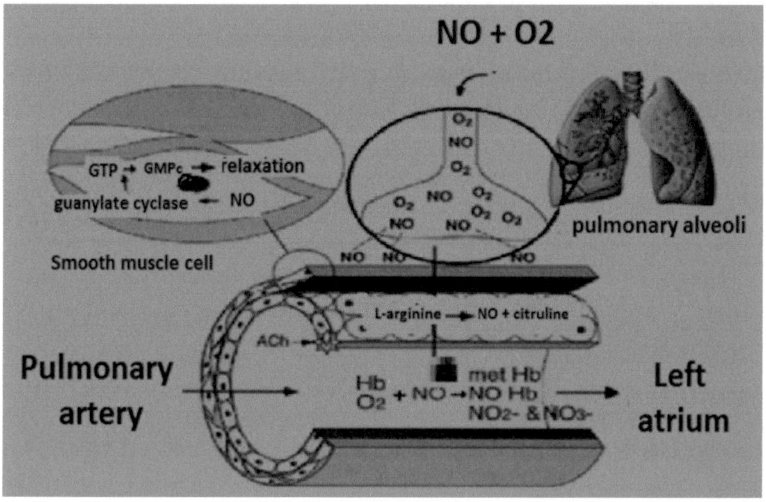

Figure 1. Schematic representation of the mechanism and site of action of inhaled nitric oxide (Adapted from Atz and Wessel [38]). Inhaled NO action, different from the NO intravenous action, is limited to veins and arteries of small resistance, and is unable to dilate large capacitance vessels. In lungs inhaled NO acts primarily on the arterial vessels but can during high venous vasoconstriction acting also in the postcapillary bed. The selective pulmonary vasodilatation produced by inhaled NO is a therapeutic option. NO binds to hemoglobin, resulting in its systemic inactivation, resulting in preservation of coronary and systemic blood pressures

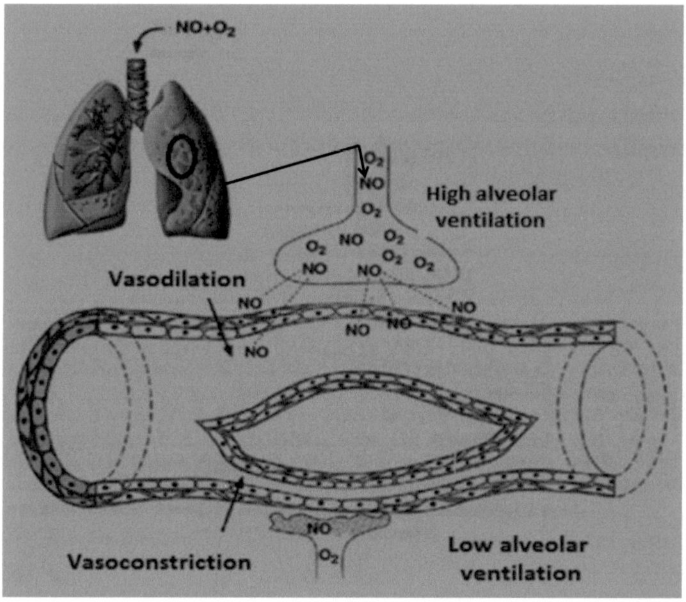

Figure 2. Schematic representation of mechanism of action in pulmonary disease (e.g.| SARA) (Adapted from Atz and Wessel [38]). In acute lung injury, inhaled NO is preferably released in areas where ventilation is high. Blood vessels are affected by the vicinity of hypoxic vasoconstriction in poorly ventilated alveoli. Inhaled NO, therefore, redirects the flow to pulmonary blood vessels dilated near well-ventilated alveoli, decreases intrapulmonary shunt and improved oxygenation

In acute lung injury, inhaled NO is preferably released in areas where ventilation is high. Blood vessels are affected by the vicinity of hypoxic vasoconstriction in poorly ventilated alveoli. Inhaled NO, therefore, redirects the flow to pulmonary blood vessels dilated near well-ventilated alveoli, decreases intrapulmonary shunt and improves oxygenation (Figure 2).

Well-defined study at INCOR in 14 adult patients with pulmonary hypertension confirmed the effect of inhaled NO, but with the caveat that pulmonary mechanics may interfere with its efficacy.[19]

2. Technical and ethical aspects

Inhaled NO in high concentrations is toxic, causing methemoglobinemia and lung injury, mainly by oxidation to NO2. International experiences have shown significant pulmonary injury vasodilatation in patients breathing low concentrations of 5-40 ppm, these levels appear not to be toxic. The 80 ppm maintained the methemoglobin levels below 3% for 3 hours. Isolated cases reported in the literature showed that the use of NO inhalation during 53 days was not associated with elevated levels of methemoglobin. Nitric oxide cannot be used intravenously because it is rapidly inactivated by hemoglobin. This makes inhaling job absolutely safe for the patient since possible excesses of the absorbed gas are "scavenged" by hemoglobin and there are subpopulations of patients with impaired ability to reduce methemoglobin.

The greatest concerns regarding the clinical use of NO are the safety of medical and paramedical staff involved in patient care due to the toxic effects of NO2. The U.S. Occupational Safety and Health Administration (OSHA) states that above 25 ppm inhaled NO is permissible in a work environment, for over 8 hours a day, with occasional increases up to 100ppm [20].

3. Critical analysis

A meta-analysis using information extracted up to 1996 from the two most prestigious banks of medical literature references (Medline and Current Contents), and data from specialized conferences, highlighted some of the key features on the use of inhaled NO. [21]

- Inhaled NO is now recognized as a valuable pharmacological tool in neonatal and pediatric intensive care medicine, surgery and cardiopulmonary disease;
- Other applications, such as chronic obstructive pulmonary disease and acute respiratory distress syndrome in adults, require careful monitoring;
- Treatment with inhaled NO is relatively inexpensive but should be used in all patients based on the paradigms of its effectiveness and potential toxicity;
- Recent discoveries of its anti-inflammatory and extrapulmonary effects open new horizons for future applications.

http://dx.doi.org/10.5772/57109

A critical analysis, although with no pretension of addressing all aspects of the use of inhaled NO in cardiac surgery, should include some questions and possible answers.

Are there advantages of using inhaled NO and/or hyperventilation to control pulmonary hypertension after surgical repair of congenital heart disease?

In principle: yes. Inhaled NO and hyperventilation are both effective in reducing pulmonary artery pressure (PAP) and pulmonary vascular resistance (PVR). However, the selective action of inhaled NO on pulmonary circulation offers advantages over hyperventilation because the decrease in cardiac output and increased systemic vascular resistance (SVR) are undesirable in the perioperative time. [22] It should be noted that NO in oxygen appears to be a more potent pulmonary vasodilator than oxygen alone. [23]

Is there any influence of inhaled NO on the survival of patients with secondary pulmonary hypertension?

Although inhaled NO can reduce pulmonary hypertension, it seems that this action is not associated with better survival. A randomized study is needed to determine the exact role of inhaled NO on the survival of patients with residual pulmonary hypertension after surgical treatment. [24] A randomized controlled study was carried out to test the hypothesis that inhaled nitric oxide (iNO) would improve the hemodynamic effects, and short-term clinical outcomes, of 29 patients with mitral stenosis and severe pulmonary hypertension, who underwent cardiac surgery [25]. The authors concluded that iNO immediately after surgery in patients with mitral stenosis and severe pulmonary hypertension improves hemodynamics and may have short-term clinical benefits. In addition, there are evidences that the postoperative co-administration of iNO and oral sildenafil in patients with out-of-proportion pulmonary hypertension undergoing cardiac surgery is safe, and resulting in an additive favorable effect on pulmonary arterial pressure and pulmonary vascular resistance, without systemic hypotension and ventilation/perfusion mismatch.[26]

Are there subgroups of congenital heart disease that can best benefit from the use of inhaled NO?

The answer is questionable. Studies have shown that inhaled NO causes minimal advantage over PAP or cardiac output (CO) in children after repair of the atrioventricular canal. [27]. More recently, clinical results have been demonstrating that iNO may improve hemodynamics and patient outcome after Fontan type procedures, suggesting that the use of iNO may be an effective therapy in this pediatric surgical setting. Even the use of iNO in pediatric heart transplantation has not been extensively studied. However, the limited evidence up to this date suggests that future clinical research in this setting may provide additional insight [28].

Is it possible to predict the need for the use of inhaled NO in the postoperative period of congenital and acquired heart disease?

Some factors have been associated as predictors of the use of inhaled NO: a) Age <1 year, Down syndrome, preoperative pulmonary hypertension and increased pulmonary vascular resistance. Using a multivariate model, it was possible to identify 73% of patients using inhaled NO. In a service that allows unrestricted use of inhaled NO, 50% of children undergoing surgery for congenital heart disease have made its use.[29]

Is the association of inhaled NO with prostacyclin possible?

There are some controversies. The combination of these vasodilators was not more potent than the single use of iloprost or inhaled NO for the control of pulmonary hypertension. [30] The Beraprost appears to be a therapeutical alternative to the use of inhaled NO. The combined use of both could be an alternative therapy without significant complications in the treatment of pulmonary hypertension in children. [31, 32, 33]

Is there a therapeutic option against pulmonary hypertension "rebound" after cessation of inhaled NO?

Dipyridamole could attenuate rebound pulmonary hypertension after cessation of inhaled NO in postoperative congenital heart disease. Dipyridamole may sustain elevations of cGMP induced by inhaled NO. Furthermore, the activity of phosphodiesterase could contribute to the acute pulmonary hypertension after discontinuation of inhaled NO. [34] Isolated studies suggest sildenafil as an option against PH "rebound" after iNO withdraw [35, 36].

What about long term toxicity studies?

Considering the potential toxicity of inhaled NO, there are no studies tracking the medium and long-term patients to their therapeutic use. These studies are scarce in the literature. Japanese study, reporting the follow-up of 65 children over a period of 2.0 to 4.3 years (mean 3.1 years), states that all children no longer needed to use oxygen. In addition, potential adverse effects, including the incidence of malignant tumors or chronic inflammation of the respiratory tract were not observed. [37]

Besides the pulmonary vascular resistance reduction, are there other effects of inhaled NO that may be evaluated from the therapeutic point of view?

Other actions of inhaled NO should raise interest in their therapeutic potential: Inhaled NO attenuates the proliferation of vascular smooth muscle, inhibits platelet aggregation, promotes cytoprotection for organ donors, improves the ischemic reperfusion injury, should develop angiogenesis in immature lungs and improve the ability to carry oxygen by hemoglobin in anemic falciform patients. [38] In addition, the emerging understanding of the systemic effects of iNO on inflammation opens potential therapeutic opportunities. [39]

Would the use of NO donor drugs and other drugs by inhalation, as an alternative to inhaled NO, be possible or reasonable?

At least one published work indicates that nitroglycerin spray is effective, cheap and safe to control pulmonary hypertension associated with congenital heart defects in services that do not have the resources of extracorporeal membrane oxygenation and/or inhaled NO. [40] In the Neonatal Intensive Care Unit of Ribeirão Preto Faculty of Medicine Hospital, sodium nitroprusside by inhalation has been used in extreme cases. Randomly, some infants had transient vasodilatation and became stained. In some cases, no effect was observed. Sodium nitroprusside was used in an adult patient with severe right ventricular dysfunction secondary to pulmonary hypertension associated to atrial septal defect and pulmonary thromboembolism. In postoperative pulmonary thromboendarterectomy, seven years after ASD correction, the levels of pulmonary hypertension reached 180 mmHg. Sodium nitroprusside intravenously decreased pulmonary arterial pressure but was associated with severe hypotension, although lower in magnitude than the intravenous route. It was not possible to conclude that the hypotension was associated to systemic absorption of nitroprusside used by inhalation. Inhaled milrinone can be an alternative to nitric oxide. A randomized clinical trial including thirty-five children below the age of 12 years who were suffering from acyanotic congenital heart disease with left-to-right intracardiac shunt and pulmonary artery hypertension (mean PA pressure > 30 mmHg) was carried out to match the acute effects of inhaled milrinone and inhaled nitroglycerin. Both inhaled drugs were effective as a valuable therapeutic option and can help reduce the high inspired oxygen concentrations needed to treat pulmonary artery hypertensive episodes in perioperative settings. [41,42]

Is there any benefit in using inhaled nitric oxide in pulmonary hypertension due to heart failure?

There are few studies that illustrate the experience with its use in congestive heart failure (CHF), which presents controversial aspects:

- In patients with CHF, the decrease in pulmonary vascular resistance is accompanied by increased values of capillary pulmonary pressure "wedge". Study of 10 patients, using 20 ppm NO inhalation, had no effect on left ventricular function, concluding that the increase of the capillary "wedge" pressure is due mainly to altered conditions of ventricular filling related to pulmonary hypertension secondary to severe CHF; [43]
- The negative inotropic effects of inhaled NO in the usual concentrations of 20 ppm are not relevant. It was determined experimentally in dogs that the increase in filling pressures seems to be secondary to the primary vasodilator effect of NO, without affecting the properties of contraction and relaxation of the left ventricle; [44.45]
- Inhaled NO would be particularly useful in the main event of isolated right ventricle failure, a less frequent situation in cases of congestive heart failure due to dilated cardiomyopathy;
- Bocchi et al., in Brazil, demonstrated that the use of inhaled NO in patients with CHF attenuated the excessive increase in tidal volume during exercise. The same authors reported the occurrence of pulmonary edema with the use of inhaled NO in patients with severe CHF. [46]

These data allow us to assert that there is no consensus for the use of inhaled NO in the treatment of pulmonary hypertension in patients with CHF. However, it can be an option in extreme and difficult to control cases, as the usual treatment. In these cases, we should be attentive to the patients worsening, and concentrations above 20 ppm are not useful. In adults with ischemic heart disease, abrupt vasodilatation may sometimes lower left ventricular filling enough to increase blood flow and dangerously increase the preload of a left ventricular function, with a possible increase of the left atrium pressure and pulmonary edema. This does not seem to be related to potential NO negative inotropic effect. [47,48,49]

Considering the reviewed aspects, which highlighted many controversies, are any conclusions possible?

One thing is certain. Arguably, although inhaled NO is a selective pulmonary vasodilator and, in no doubt, will save lives, its use has not become unanimity in a period of more than 10 years. This is certainly due to its potential toxicity and response variability (observed even in neonatology), facts that do not support the realization of large trials, which could explain many of the mentioned controversies.

In the early 90s, one of the authors (PRBE) visited cardinal U.S. clinics (Mayo Clinic, Cleveland Clinic, Johns Hopkins and Harvard) which began clinical trials with inhaled NO. A summary of these clinical observations and interviews stressed the following:

- The effectiveness of treatment in individual cases;
- The variability of response to treatment regardless of age, heart and / or respiratory disease;
- Improved therapeutic response, although transient, were observed in the most significant hypertensions and chronic lung;
- The belief that inhaled NO would be a potential therapeutic tool that could benefit transient hypertensions in neonatology and cardiopulmonary transplants;
- All physicians showed concern about NO potential toxicity, not only to patients, but also to the professional health team.
- It seems that, after decades, these observations are still present and relevant. Only one standard agreement about the use of lower doses (10-20 ppm) then originally used.

A meta-analysis of the references cited in Medline until 2002, illustrates the evolution and current role of inhaled NO in cardiac surgery. When comparing the total number of published studies/articles with the number of studies in humans, it is observed that the majority (71.36%) is related to humans. When inhaled NO is associated with pulmonary hypertension, it is observed a total number of references relative to 43.32% of the total, with prevalence of about 57.04% of human studies. When inhaled NO is associated as part of the therapeutic arsenal of ARDS, the total number of studies corresponds to 9.9% of the total, with prevalence of about 78% of studies in humans. When inhaled NO is associated as part of therapeutic heart failure, the total number of studies corresponds to 5.1% of the total, with prevalence of about 86.25% of studies in humans. [50]

Observing the *Web of Science* the data, pulmonary hypertension is still the primary target for the inhaled NO therapeutic use (44.5%). There is a decreased interest in the investigations on the applicability in ARDS, and the human studies are strongly prevalent (Figure 3).

When searching for studies, again until 2002, related specifically to therapeutic use of NO in cardiac surgery, the number of publications is about 2.5% of the total. When considering the therapeutic use of inhaled NO not only concerning cardiac surgery in general, but also including valve heart disease, congenital heart disease, heart transplant and lung transplant, the total number of communications is around 320. Of these publications, 14.7% corresponds to cardiac surgery in general, 27.6% to the heart valve, 12.5% to heart transplantation, 37% to congenital heart defects and 29.5% to lung transplants. [50]

Nowadays, the updated number of publications specifically to therapeutic use of NO in cardiac surgery is of about 3.5% of the total. Considering valve heart disease, congenital heart disease and heart transplant surgeries, the total number of communications is around 290. Of these publications, heart valve diseases corresponds to 4.8%, heart transplantation to 20.0% and congenital heart defects to 31, 4% (Figure 4).

http://dx.doi.org/10.5772/57109

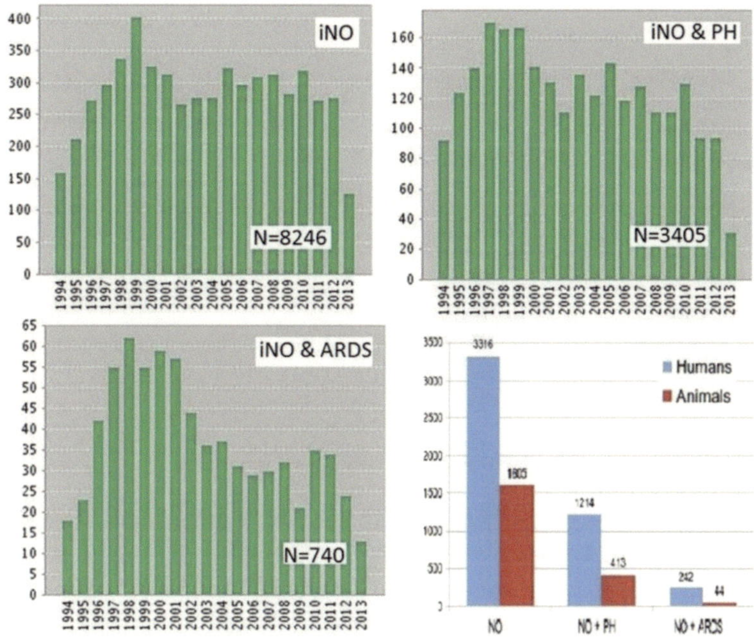

Figure 3. Graphical representation of the number of Thomson Reuters (formerly ISI) Web of Knowledge references.

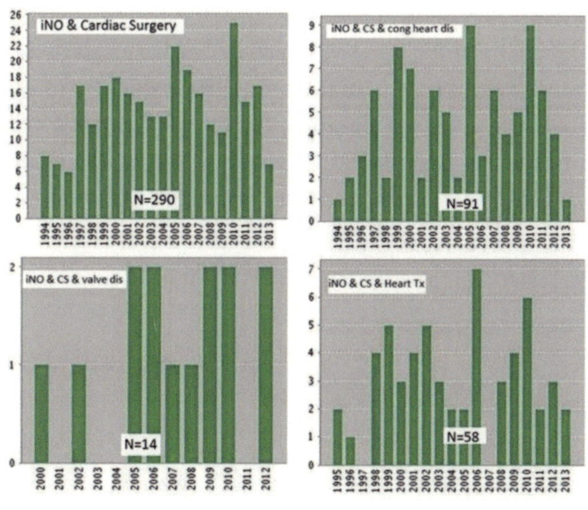

Figure 4. Graphical representation of the number of Thomson Reuters (formerly ISI) Web of Knowledge references.

In a period of 20 years (1990-2010), there was a marked drop in the number of publications regarding the use of iNO in heart transplant. This number remained below 3% for cases of coronary artery bypass graft, around 15% for publications on the use of iNO in surgeries for heart valve disease treatment (tendency to decrease) and congenital heart disease (tendency to increase) (Figure 5).

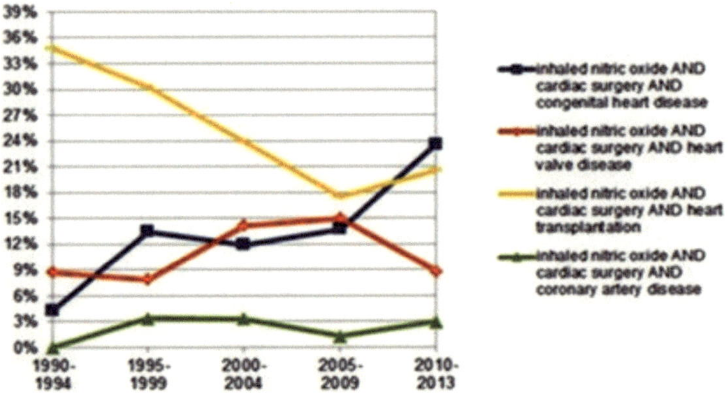

Figure 5. Graphical representation of the timeline decades of MEDLINE references

The apparent decrease of iNO use in surgeries to correct congenital cardiac defects highlights some doubts about its real usefulness. Cochrane Database System Review observed no differences in the use of iNO when compared to control in the majority of outcomes reviewed. No data were available for analysis concerning several clinical outcomes, including long-term mortality and neurodevelopmental outcome. The authors found it difficult to draw valid conclusions because of concerns regarding methodological quality, bias, sample size, and heterogeneity. [51]

These data confirm the observations and trends regarding the future therapeutic use of inhaled NO. Its use is not made unanimously, and the groups that are most benefited are those in which pulmonary hypertension is transient. Considering the relatively small number of reports, many associated with isolated cases, and a prominent prevalence of human observation, more experimental investigations are needed. Perhaps this fact is due partly to the difficulty of obtaining appropriate experimental models of pulmonary hypertension, but obviously due to the unknown about potential long-term toxic effects of inhaled NO. In the absence of trials involving large numbers of patients, and despite its potential toxicity, inhaled NO should be used, with extraordinary technical accuracy, as a therapeutic test that can save lives.

4. Concluding remarks

A Societad Iberoamericana de Información Scientific (SIIC) and a Brazilian Journal of Cardiovascular Surgery reports, in 2002, motivated the current review [50]. Updating the data so far, it can be said that the outlook for the use of inhaled NO changed little or nothing. It is worth mentioning a recent meta-analysis clinical trial for a real assessment of the problem, which was based in The Cochrane Central Register of Controlled Trials, and the reviewers support the following conclusions [51,52]:

- Inhaled NO shows no effect on mortality and improves oxygenation transiently in patients with hypoxemic respiratory failure,

- The lack of information does not allow the assessment of other clinically relevant goals,
- New trials comparing inhaled NO with some inhaled placebo will be essential to stratify the primary disease and assess the impact of other forms of combination therapy for respiratory failure
- They will need estimate, specifically, effects before any clinically relevant benefit of inhaled NO for respiratory failure can be excluded.

Author details

Alfredo José Rodrigues[1], Patricia Martinez Evora[2] and Paulo Roberto Barbosa Evora[1]

1 Department of Surgery and Anatomy, Ribeirão Preto School of Medicine, University of São Paulo, Brazil

2 School of Agricultural and Veterinary Sciences at Jaboticabal, São Paulo State University, Brazil

References

[1] Furchgott RF & Zawadzki JV. The obligatory role of endothelial cells in the relaxation of arterial smooth muscle by acetylcholine. Nature 1980, 288: 373-6.

[2] Cherry PD, Furchgott RF, Zawadzki JV, D. Jothianandan. Role of endothelial cells in relaxation of isolated arteries by bradykinin. Proc Natl Acad Sci USA 1982, 79:2106-10.

[3] Cocks T & Angus JA. Bioassay of the release of endothelium-derived relaxing factor (EDRF) from isolated endothelial cells in vitro. In: Bevan JA, Godfraind T, Maxwell RA, Stoclet JS, Worcel M, eds. Vascular neuroeffector mechanisms. Amsterdam: Elsevier, 1985:131-6.

[4] Furchgott RF. Studies on relaxation of rabbit aorta by sodium nitrite: the basis for the Proposal That the acid-activated inhibitory factor from bovine retractor penis is inorganic nitrite and the endothelium-derived relaxing factor is nitric oxide. In: Vanhoutte PM, ed. Mechanisms of vasodilatation. New York: Raven Press, 1988:401-14. Vol. IV.

[5] Ignarro LJ, Byrns RE, Wood KS. Biochemical and pharmacological properties of EDRF and Its similarity to nitric oxide radical. In: Vanhoutte PM, ed. Mechanisms of vasodilatation. New York: Raven Press, 1988:427-35. Vol. IV.

[6] Palmer RM, Ferrige AG, Moncada S. Nitric oxide release accounts for the biological activity of endothelium-derived relaxing factor. Nature 1987, 327:524-6.

[7] Palmer MR Ashton DS, Moncada S. Vascular endothelial cells synthesize nitric oxide from L-arginine. Nature 1988, 333:664-6.

[8] Frostell C, Fratacci MD, Wain JC, Jones R, Zapol WM. Inhaled nitric oxide: a selective pulmonary vasodilator reversing hypoxic pulmonary vasoconstriction. Circulation 1991, 83:2038-47.

[9] Moncada S, Palmer RM, Higgs EA. Nitric oxide: physiology, pathophysiology, and pharmacology. Pharmacol Rev 1991, 43:109-42.

[10] Snyder SH, Bredt DS. Biological roles of nitric oxide. Sci Am 1992, 266:68-77.

[11] AP Tavares Pimenta Junior AG, Evora PR. Basis for the therapeutic use of inhaled nitric oxide. Arq Bras Cardiol 1995, 64:45-52.

[12] Frostell CG, Blomqvist H, Hedenstierna G, J Lundberg, Zapol WM. Inhaled nitric oxide selectively reverses human hypoxic pulmonary vasoconstriction Causing without systemic vasodilatation. Anesthesiology 1993; 78:427-35.

[13] Wessel DL, Adatia I, Giglia TM, Thompson JE, Kulik TJ. Use of inhaled nitric oxide and acetylcholine in the evaluation of pulmonary hypertension and endothelial function after cardiopulmonary bypass. Circulation 1993, 88 (5 pt 1), 2128-38.

[14] Roberts JD, Jr., Lang P Bigatello LM, GJ Vlahakes, Zapol WM. Inhaled nitric oxide in congenital heart disease. Circulation 1993, 87:447-53.

[15] Vallance P, J Collier, Moncada S. Effects of endothelium-derived nitric oxide on peripheral arteriolar tone in man. Lancet 1989; 2:997-1000.

[16] Cremona G, Dinh-Xuan AT, Higenbottam TW. Endothelium-derived relaxing factor and the pulmonary circulation. Lung 1991, 169:185-202.

[17] Roos CM, Rich GF, Uncles DR, Daugherty MO, Frank DU. Sites of vasodilatation by inhaled nitric oxide vs. sodium nitroprusside in endothelin-constricted isolated rat lungs. J Appl Physiol 1994, 77:51-7.

[18] Benzing A Geiger & K. Inhaled nitric oxide lowers pulmonary capillary pressure and changes longitudinal distribution of pulmonary vascular resistance in Patients with acute lung injury. Acta Anaesthesiol Scand 1994; 38:640-5.

[19] Carmona MJ & Auler Jr. OJ. Effects of inhaled nitric oxide on respiratory system mechanics, Hemodynamics, and gas exchange after cardiac surgery. J Vasc Cardiothorac Anesth 1998, 12:157-61.

[20] Centers for Disease Control. Recommendation for occupational safety and health standard. MMWR Morb Mortal Wkly Rep 1980; 37: S7.

[21] Troncy E, M Francoeur, Blaise G. Inhaled nitric oxide: clinical applications, Indications, and toxicology. Can J Anaesth 1997, 44:973-88.

[22] Morris K, M Beghetti, Petros A, Adatia I, Bohn D. Comparison of hyperventilation and inhaled nitric oxide for pulmonary hypertension after repair of congenital heart disease. Crit Care Med 2000; 28:2974-8.

[23] KG Allman, JD Young, Carapiet D, Stevens JE, Ostman-Smith I, Archer LN. Effects of oxygen and nitric oxide in oxygen on pulmonary arterial Pressures of children with congenital cardiac defects. Pediatr Cardiol 1996; 17:246-50.

[24] Sharma R, rooted N, SK Choudhary et al. Does inhaled nitric oxide Improve survival in operated congenital disease with severe pulmonary hypertension? Indian Heart J 2001, 53:48-55.

[25] ernandes JL, Sampaio RO, Brandão CM, Accorsi TA, Cardoso LF, Spina GS, Tarasoutchi F, Pomerantzeff P, Auler JO Jr, Grinberg M. Comparison of inhaled nitric oxide versus oxygen on hemodynamics in patients with mitral stenosis and severe pulmonary hypertension after mitral valve surgery. Am J Cardiol. 2011;107:1040-5.

[26] Matamis D, Pampori S, Papathanasiou A, Papakonstantinou P, Tsagourias M, Galiatsou E, Koulouras V, Nakos G. Inhaled NO and sildenafil combination in cardiac surgery patients with out-of-proportion pulmonary hypertension: acute effects on postoperative gas exchange and hemodynamics. Circ Heart Fail. 2012;5:47-53.

[27] Checchia PA, Bronicki RA, Goldstein B. Review of inhaled nitric oxide in tem pediatric cardiac surgery setting. Pediatr Cardiol. 2012;33:493-505.

[28] Curran RD, Mavroudis C, Backer CL, Sautel M, Zales VR, Wessel DL. Inhaled nitric oxide for children with congenital heart disease and pulmonary hypertension. Ann Thorac Surg 1995; 60:1765-71.

[29] Laitinen PO, Rasanen J, Sairanen H. Postoperative nitric oxide therapy in children with congenital heart disease: can the need be predicted? Scand J Cardiovasc 2000, 34:149-53.

[30] Durongpisitkul K, Laoprasitiporn D, Layangool T, Sittiwankul R, Panamonta M, Mokrapong P; Thailand Multicenter Study. Comparison of the acute pulmonary vasodilating effect of beraprost sodium and nitric oxide in congenital heart disease. Circ J. 2005;69:61-4.

[31] Preston IR, Sagliani KD, Roberts KE, Shah AM, Desouza SA, Howard W, Brennan J, Hill NS. Comparison of acute hemodynamic effects of inhaled nitric oxide and inhaled epoprostenol in patients with pulmonary hypertension. Pulm Circ. 2013;3(1): 68-73.

[32] Rimensberger PC, Spahr-Schopfer I, Berner M et al. Inhaled nitric oxide versus aerosolized iloprost in secondary pulmonary hypertension in children with congenital

heart disease: vasodilator capacity and cellular mechanisms. Circulation 2001; 103:544-8.

[33] Ichida F, ESEU K, Hashimoto I et al. Acute effect of oral prostacyclin and inhaled nitric oxide on pulmonary hypertension in children. J Cardiol 1997; 29:217-24.

[34] Ivy DD, Kinsella JP, Ziegler JW, Abman SH. Dipyridamole attenuates rebound pulmonary hypertension after inhaled nitric oxide withdrawal in postoperative congenital heart disease. J Thorac Cardiovasc Surg 1998; 115:875-82.

[35] Lee JE, Hillier SC, Knoderer CA. Use of sildenafil to facilitate weaning from inhaled nitric oxide in children with pulmonary hypertension following surgery for congenital heart disease. J Intensive Care Med. 2008;23:329-34.

[36] Nakatsu T, Nemoto S, Ikeda T, Saji Y, Nakajima H, Nishina T, Ohno N, Komeda M. Prophylactic treatment of oral sildenafil citrate for pulmonary hypertension in an infant treated with inhaled nitric oxide after open-heart surgery]. Kyobu Geka. 2005;58:1136-9.

[37] Yahagi N, Kumon K Tanigami H et al. Cardiac surgery and inhaled nitric oxide: Indication and follow-up (2-4 years). Artif Organs 1998, 22:886-91.

[38] Atz AM &Wessel DL. Nitric oxide inhalation. In: Rubanyi GM, ed. Pathophysiology and clinical applications of nitric oxide. Netherlands: Harwood Academic Publishers, 1999, 471-503.

[39] Checchia PA, Bronicki RA, Goldstein B. Review of inhaled nitric oxide in the pediatric cardiac surgery setting. Pediatr Cardiol. 2012;33:493-505.

[40] Omar HA, Gong F, Sun MY, Einzig S. Nebulized nitroglycerin in children with pulmonary hypertension secondary to congenital heart disease. W V J Med 1999; 95:74-5.

[41] Denault AY, Lamarche Y, Couture P, Haddad F, Lambert J, Tardif JC, Perrault LP. Inhaled milrinone: a new alternative in cardiac surgery? Semin Cardiothorac Vasc Anesth. 2006 ;10:346-60.

[42] Singh R, Choudhury M, Saxena A, Kapoor PM, Juneja R, Kiran U. Inhaled nitroglycerin versus inhaled milrinone in children with congenital heart disease suffering from pulmonary artery hypertension. J Cardiothorac Vasc Anesth. 2010;24:797-801.]

[43] Hayward CS, Kalnins WV, Rogers P, Feneley MP, Macdonald PS, Kelly RP. Left ventricular chamber function During inhaled nitric oxide in Patients with dilated cardiomyopathy. J Cardiovasc Pharmacol. 1999, 34:749-54.

[44] Hare JM, Shernan SK Body SC Graydon E, Colucci WS, GS Couper. Influence of inhaled nitric oxide on systemic flow and ventricular filling pressure in Patients receiving mechanical circulatory assistance. Circulation. 6 1997, 95:2250-3.

[45] E Loh, EB Lankford, DJ Polidori, EB Doering-Lubit, Hanson CW, Acker MA. Cardiovascular effects of inhaled nitric oxide in a canine model of cardiomyopathy. Ann Thorac Surg. 1999, 67:1380-5.

[46] Bocchi EA, Bacal F, Auler Junior JO, Carmona MJ, Bellotti G, Pileggi F. Inhaled nitric oxide leading to pulmonary edema in stable severe heart failure. Am J Cardiol. 1994, 74:70-2.

[47] Hayward CS, Rogers P, Keogh AM, Kelly R, Spratt PM, Macdonald PS. Inhaled nitric oxide in cardiac failure: vascular versus ventricular effects. J Cardiovasc Pharmacol. 1996; 27:80-5.53

[48] Semigran MJ, Cockrill BA, Kacmarek R, Thompson BT, Zapol WM, Dec GW, Fifer MA. Hemodynamic effects of inhaled nitric oxide in heart failure. J Am Coll Cardiol. 1994, 24:982-8.

[49] AndLoh, Stamler JS, Hare JM, Loscalzo J, Colucci WS. Cardiovascular effects of inhaled nitric oxide in Patients with left ventricular dysfunction. Circulation. 1994, 90:2780-5.

[50] Evora PRB, Viaro F, Oshiro MS, Souza DG. The utilization of inhaled nitric oxide in cardiac surgery: critical analysis and actualization. Rev. Bras. Cir. Cardiovasc, 17:221-229, 2002.

[51] Bizzarro M, Gross I. Inhaled nitric oxide for the postoperative management of pulmonary hypertension in infants and children with congenital heart disease. Cochrane Database Syst Rev. 2005 Oct 19;(4):CD005055.

[52] Sokol J, Jacobs SE, Bohn D. Inhaled nitric oxide for acute hypoxemic respiratory failure in children and adults. Cochrane Database Syst Rev. 2003; CD002787.

Chapter 7

Mechanical Complications of Acute Myocardial Infarction

Luís Augusto Palma Dallan,
Luiz Roberto Palma Dallan,
Luiz Augusto Ferreira Lisboa and
Luís Alberto Oliveira Dallan

Additional information is available at the end of the chapter

http://dx.doi.org/10.5772/57110

1. Introduction

Patients with acute myocardial infarction (AMI) may have hemodynamic, electrical or mechanical complications. The acute mechanical complications are serious events with worse prognosis. When the AMI evolves into a mechanical complication, surgical therapy is mandatory, in order to decrease the high mortality in this group of patients [4].

The main mechanical complications of acute myocardial infarction correspond to: 1 - Ventricular free wall rupture, 2 - Ventricular septal rupture, 3 - Mitral regurgitation with or without ischemic papillary muscle rupture and 4 - Left ventricular aneurysm (a 2, 7).

The mechanical complications of AMI are responsible for approximately 25,000 deaths per year in the United States [8]. The ISIS-2 study showed an increased occurrence of ventricular rupture associated with thrombolytic therapy, especially in the first 24 hours of AMI and when thrombolysis had a late administration. This is due to transformation of ischemic to hemorrhagic infarction and therefore easier to rupture. [19]

However, with the advent of early thrombolytic therapy and primary coronary angioplasty, which reduced ischemia and the size of the myocardial infarction, it is estimated that this incidence has decreased in the last two decades. [7] The incidence of these diseases can be seen in Table 1.

	Ventricularfreewallrupture	Ventricular Septum Rupture	IschemicPapillaryMuscle Rupture	Left Ventrícular Aneurysm
Prevalence	1-3% without reperfusion therapy, 3,9% in cardiogenic shock	0,8 - 6,2%	1%, greater incidence in the post-medial papillary muscle rupture	5 a 38%, greater incidence in anterior AMI
Reduction with early reperfusion	Yes	Yes	Yes	Yes

Table 1. Incidence of major mechanical complications of acute myocardial infarction [1, 2, 3, 6, 19]

In table 2 are shown the most frequent sites of rupture in fatal cases of mechanical complications after AMI.

Site	Rupture Incidence (%)
Free Ventricular wall	85
Ventricular Septum	10
Pappilary muscle	5

Table 2. Most frequent sites of rupture in fatal cases of mechanical complications after AMI. [7]

Mechanical defects usually occur in the first two weeks after AMI, with bimodal incidence, especially in the first 24 hours of AMI and after 3-5 days of its inception.

The diagnosis should be suspected whenever a patient shows signs and symptoms of hemodynamic instability, and can be established with precision from the transthoracic or transesophageal echocardiography. Pulmonary artery catheterization and monitoring of hemodynamic parameters can also be useful for detecting the defect and to guide their approach. [1, 3]

Surgical evaluation should be performed early whenever there is suspicion of a mechanical complication. Surgical treatment of emergency / urgency is indicated in most cases because the clinical treatment alone is related to high mortality rates [1, 3].

2. Diagnosis

The early diagnosis and intervention are important in trying to alter the course of an adverse outcome of patients with mechanical complications after AMI.

For the diagnosis of mechanical complications, it is necessary high degree of clinical suspicion. Besides the physical examination, imaging tests such as two-dimensional echocardiography and color Doppler are useful and practical, since they have high specificity and can be performed at bedside. Transesophageal echocardiography may improve the diagnostic accuracy in these cases [7].

Diagnosis can also be confirmed by passing a Swan-Ganz catheter, which can result in an increase in the venous blood oxygenation in the case of ventricular septal defect, as shown in Table 3:

	Ventricularfreewallrupture	Ventricular Septum Rupture	IschemicPapillaryMuscle Rupture
Main findings in central catheterization	Clinical signs of cardiac tamponade may be seen (equalization of diastolic pressures between the heart chambers)	"Oximetric jump": Increase in oxygen saturation between the right atrium and the pulmonary artery, forming "Ventricular Shunt" Large "V" waves	No oximetric jump in the right ventricle; Presence of significant large "V" waves; high values of pulmonary capillary pressure

Table 3. Main findings in Swan-Ganz catheterization [2, 3]

More than half of the patients with ventricular rupture or papillary muscle have coronary artery disease in other arteries besides the charge of the infarcted area. Therefore, whenever possible, there should be performed coronary angiography to identify other lesions that requires surgical repair, avoiding further episodes of occlusion that would increase mortality [3, 7].

3. Clinical treatment

Clinical treatment should be instituted early in all cases of mechanical complications after AMI, and ideally should be carried out intensively in specific units such as Intensive Care Unit or Coronary Care Units. Inotropes and vasodilators should be used to ensure hemodynamic stabilization for subsequent surgical treatment [1].

The Swan-Ganz catheter brings important hemodynamic information, guiding the hydration and the administration of vasoactive drugs. In cases of ventricular rupture and cardiogenic shock originating from the right ventricle infarction, aggressive volume replacement is essential for the survival of the patient.

The use of ventricular assist with the insertion of intra-aortic balloon, particularly in patients with acute mitral regurgitation or ventricular septal rupture, helps stabilize the patient, preparing him for surgery.

4. Main mechanical complications

4.1. Ventricular free wall rupture (VFWR)

4.1.1. Incidence and evolution

The incidence of ventricular free wall rupture (VFWR) in AMIs varies between 0.8-6.2%. It occurs in about 10-24% of patients who die due to AMI and represents 85% of deaths from myocardial rupture. Thus, it is the third leading cause of death, surpassed only by cardiogenic shock and the ventricular arrhythmias. [2, 9, 10]

About 30% of cardiac ruptures occur within the first 24 hours after infarction. VFWR is also observed more frequently in women, elderly, during the first episode of AMI, and in patients with previous heart attacks.

It is seven times more frequent in the left ventricle than the right ventricle, and in most cases is associated with extensive transmural infarction, with involvement of the anterior or lateral territory irrigation of left anterior descending artery. [2, 11, 17]

Other factors that increase the incidence of heart failure are hypertension during the acute phase of infarction, lack of collateral circulation, absence of chest pain, associated mitral regurgitation, Q waves on ECG, the use of corticosteroids or non-steroidal anti-inflammatory and the use of fibrinolytic agents after more than 14 hours of symptom onset or when fibrinolytic therapy is ineffective. [3, 12]

4.1.2. Symptoms

The rupture can be complete, leading to severe hemopericardium and its consequences that usually result in death due to cardiac tamponade. It may also be incomplete, which occurs when a thrombus or a hematoma, together with the pericardium, seal the ventricular free wall lesion, avoiding hemopericardium and forming a pseudoaneurysm. [2]

The main clinical findings may be manifested by characteristic chest pain of angina, pericardial or pleuritic pain, syncope, hypotension, arrhythmias, nausea, fatigue, or sudden death. Physical examination may reveal jugular stasis [29%), paradoxical pulse (47%), electromechanical dissociation and cardiogenic shock. [3]

The main clinical manifestations of rupture of ventricular free wall, according to their type, are shown in table 4:

Acute	Massive hemorrhage, electromechanical dissociation; sudden death
Subacute	Moderate hemorrhage, cardiac tamponade, cardiogenic shock
Cronic	Minor hemorrhage, false aneurysm formation, heart failure

Table 4. The main clinical manifestations of rupture of ventricular free wall [4]

4.1.3. Diagnosis

The main electrocardiographic signs that can be observed are the preservation and increase of ST segment elevation in more than one derivation and sudden variations of the T wave, or the presence of ST segment elevation in aVL, prior to rupture, with rapid progression to collapse hemodynamic and electro-mechanical dissociation. It may be further evidenced sinus tachycardia and / or ST segment elevation in V5 and may be predictive of inferior wall myocardial infarction. [2]

The Swan-Ganz catheter data may show classic signs of cardiac tamponade (equalization of diastolic pressures between the heart chambers).

Echocardiography can demonstrate pericardial effusion greater than 5 mm, increased echotexture of the pericardial contents (blood clot), direct visualization of the lesion or signs of cardiac tamponade. [3]. In subacute or chronic cases, in addition to echocardiography, magnetic resonance imaging of the heart may help both to confirm the diagnosis and the orientation of the best surgical approach.

4.1.4. Surgical treatment

In most cases, surgical treatment is an emergency. Pericardial drainage can be performed for relief of cardiac tamponade before surgical correction. In this case, the patient should be prepared for cannulation and extracorporeal circulation, to prevent hemodynamic collapse. [12, 13]

The mortality of complete ventricular rupture is approximately 100%, and that surgical treatment reduces this ratio to values around 60%. [1, 2, 3]. Surgical treatment involves ventricular suture directly or with a patch to cover the ventricular perforation, always associated with revascularization when possible. The use of biological adhesives such as cyanoacrylate has been made to fix the patch around the necrotic tissue. [1, 12, 13]

Among the surgical techniques are: [1, 2, 12, 13]

- Infarctectomy and suturing the edges anchored in Teflon patch;
- Sutures of a large patch covering the infarcted area to fix the break;
- Use of a Teflon patch covering the infarcted area with use of biological glue.

In cases of subacute rupture with thrombus formation and spontaneous control of hemorrhage, there is an opportunity of the initial clinical treatment with stabilization and control of cardiogenic shock. In this situation the patient will be operated in better clinical conditions and consequently will improve surgical outcomes. However, the surgical indication must be to prevent premature rupture of the ventricle. [1]

The incomplete rupture of ventricular free wall, or also called "pseudo breaks" with false aneurysm formation, are more benign forms of presentation of this serious disease. In these cases, intensive medical therapy with hemodynamic control shows good initial results. The indication for surgery is delayed for 15 to 30 days after the acute phase of infarction, a period that has already begun to form myocardial fibrosis facilitating the surgical approach.

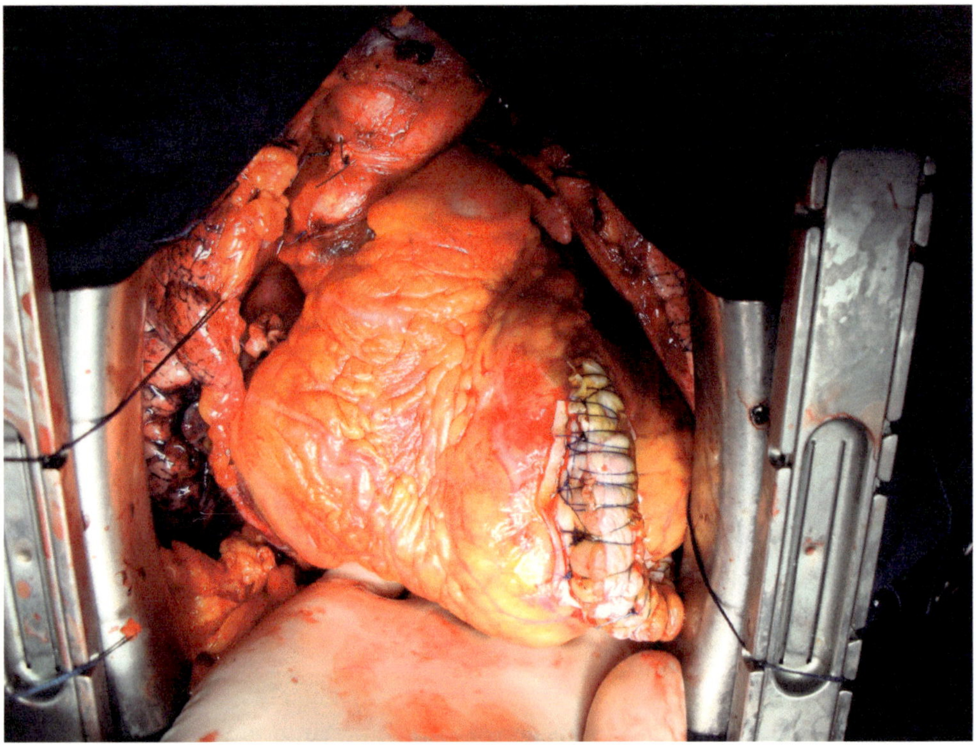

Figure 1. Surgical repair of acute left ventricular rupture

4.2. Ventricular septum rupture (VSR)

4.2.1. Incidence and evolution

The incidence of ventricular septal rupture (VSR) has declined since the beginning of fibrinolytic era, and reduced from 1-3% to 0.2%-0.3% with coronary reperfusion, as evidenced by the large GUSTO-I study.

Although there is an increased risk of ventricular rupture with the use of fibrinolytics, the early reperfusion and the decrease of the extention of the necrotic area are responsible for reducing the incidence of mechanical complications in such cases. [15]

It occurs most frequently between 3-7 days after AMI when recanalization therapy has not being done. [16] The mortality of VSR stays around 94%, while that in patients who underwent surgical treatment it is around 20-60% [1, 2, 3]

4.2.2. Symptoms

The main clinical findings may be manifested by rough holosystolic murmur in the region of the left lower sternal border, usually associated with clinical worsening of the patient, accentuated second heart sound, pulmonary edema, signs of right or left ventricular failure and cardiogenic shock. [2]

4.2.3. Diagnosis

The electrocardiogram is not specific. Echocardiography may show ventricular septal defect, left-right shunt on color Doppler through the septum, signs of right ventricular overload. Coronary angiography and cardiac catheterization confirmed the VSD and the coronary lesions. [2, 3] The data of the Swan-Ganz catheter may show an “oximetric jump”, characterized by an increase in oxygen saturation between the right atrium and the pulmonary artery, forming the "Ventricular Shunt." In addition, waves can be observed "V" large.

4.2.4. Surgical treatment

Before surgery some essential cares should be performed, such as invasive monitoring, treatment with anti-arrhythmic drugs, inotropes, vasodilators and the passage of intra-aortic balloon in unstable patients.

The hemodynamic treatment of ventricular septal defect has been studied through the VSD closure with devices installed percutaneously. However, surgery remains the treatment of choice so far, mainly due to the small number of patients studied and lack of data that provides meaningful results and secure the new technique.

The urgent surgical treatment should be instituted in all patients, even those with preserved ventricular function, who do not have pulmonary edema or cardiogenic shock. Hemodynamic collapse even sudden death may happen, because the ventricular impaired location can suddenly expand the tissue stress and rupture [1, 3]

The earlier the surgery is performed, the better is the evolution of the patient. The techniques for surgical correction of this complication include: [1, 2, 7]

- Use of biological tissue preserved, with or without infarctectomy and aneurysmectomy;
- Apical amputation technique to correct the defect in this portion of the ventricle;
- Plication to repair the rupture in the anterior-septal;
- Use of Dacron or bovine pericardium endocardial and epicardial suture to support;
- Correction of posterior septal rupture using the pericardium in a "sandwich", including the septal defect and ventriculotomy;
- Use of biological glue such as cyanoacrylate.

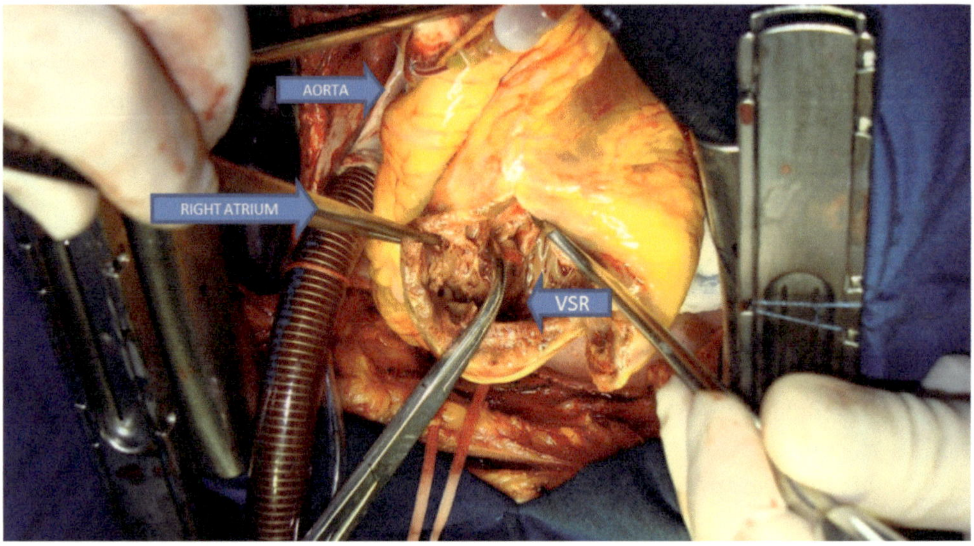

Figure 2. Ventricular septal rupture (VSR) accessed through anterior ventricular infartected free wall

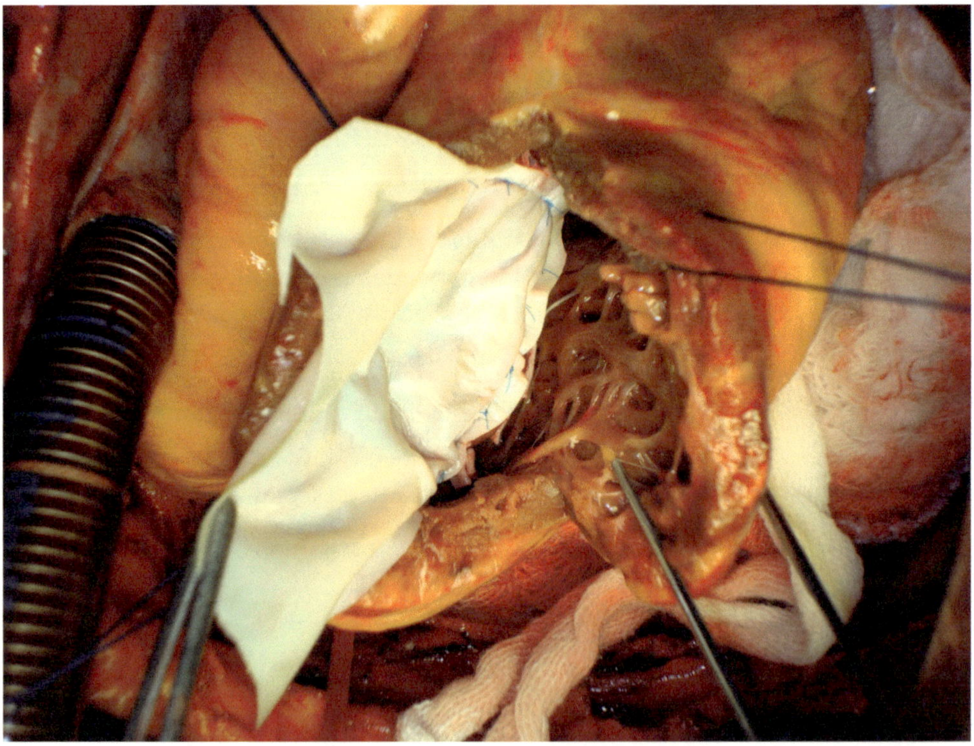

Figure 3. Ventricular septal rupture repair with the use of bovine pericardium

4.3. Mitral valve regurgitation with or without papillary muscle rupture (MVR)

4.3.1. Incidence and Evolution

Mitral valve regurgitation (MVR) occurs mainly in patients with inferior AMI, leading to extreme instability when associated with papillary muscle rupture, even in patients with moderate coronary heart disease.

The most frequently affected papillary muscle is the postero-medial, since the posterior interventricular artery or the circumflex artery are the only responsables for it's irrigation. [1, 2, 14]

The MVR typically occurs in the first two weeks after AMI, with bimodal incidence, especially in the first 24 hours of AMI and after 3-5 days of its inception.

MVR associated with cardiogenic shock carries a poor prognosis. In the SHOCK study, approximately 10% of CABG patients had severe shock, and had a mortality rate of 55%. In the SAVE study, in which patients were treated with inhibitors of angiotensin-converting enzyme after AMI, even patients with mild mitral insufficiency had worse prognosis compared to those without valvular dysfunction. [3, 16]

When complete papillary muscle rupture happens, even with surgical intervention, the mortality rate is high [30-70%), and some factors such as extent of infarction, cardiogenic shock, patient´s age and delayed operatory indication increase this index. [4]

4.3.2. Symptoms

Mitral regurgitation may have different degrees of importance, from mild and even asymptomatic, which are usually incidental findings of tests such as echocardiography and catheterization, to severe, with hemodynamic instability evident.

The clinical picture may be manifested by abrupt establishment of dyspnea and pulmonary edema associated with hypotension. The physical examination may show systolic murmur in the mitral regurgitation, and signs of right ventricular hypertrophy, severe pulmonary edema and cardiogenic shock. [3]

4.3.3. Diagnosis

The electrocardiogram is not characteristic. The echocardiogram may show left ventricular dyskinesia, papillary muscle or injury of the chordae tendineae and severe mitral valve regurgitation by Doppler color. Moreover, it can quantify the degree of valvular insufficiency. [2, 3]

Swan-Ganz parameters shows the presence of "V" wave and significant pulmonary capillary wedge pressure, but not an increase variation on oxigen saturation at the right ventricle, confirming the mitral regurgitation and excluding the presence of ventricular septal defect.

Coronary angiography and ventriculography shows clearly the mitral regurgitation.

4.3.4. Surgical treatment

Treatment will be established according to patient´s hemodynamic stability. Treated clinically, only 25% of patients survive the first 24 hours after rupture of the papillary muscle. The median survival without surgical treatment is three days, and several authors consider the complete rupture of the papillary muscle of the body as incompatible with life. [1] On the other hand, discrete mitral regurgitation is generally treated with oral medications at first.

Invasive monitoring and the use of inotropic and vasodilators should be considered in severe cases, in order to reduce left ventricle´s afterload and to reduce mitral regurgitation.

Intra-aortic balloon is required in the most unstable patients. The high mortality rate is related to significant hemodynamic compromise with cardiogenic shock preoperatively. [2, 3]

It is observed lower mortality in mitral valve repair [13%) compared to its replacement [47.4%). [1, 14]

In cases of valve replacement, mortality is related to resection of the papillary muscle, with reported benefits of its preservation. The intraoperative transesophageal echocardiography has improved the surgical results by avoiding residual defects. [2]

Another often surgical procedure mitral valve annuloplasty, and it should be performed concomitantly with CABG when possible. In such cases, the distal anastomosis of the grafts to the coronary arteries should be performed before valve replacement. [1, 14]

4.4. Left ventricular aneurysm (LVA)

4.4.1. Incidence and evolution

Left ventricular aneurysm is a serious complication of AMI, and its incidence ranges from 5 to 38%. The LVA usually occurs in the left anterior ventricle wall, associated with complete occlusion of the left anterior descending artery, and it is four times more frequent than in inferior wall infarction. [2]

AMI patients undergoing fibrinolytic therapy whith early recanalization have a significant reduction in the incidence of ventricular aneurysm (7.2%) compared to those not receiving fibrinolytics (18.8%). [3]

Several factors are involved in the formation of AV, as the extent of necrotic area, absence of collateral circulation and pathophysiology of ventricular remodeling. The AV is found in approximately 10-15% of survivors of AMI, with the rate six times higher in patients with AV than in those without aneurysm. [2]

These aneurysms are more prevalent among males, in the proportion of 2.2 to 1. Its incidence ranges from 45 to 74 years old, corresponding to the highest incidence of AMI.

The mortality is approximately 49% corresponding to 65-80% in those formed in the earlier stages and 23% formed in the later stages of the myocardial infarction.

4.4.2. Symptoms

The symptoms may be manifested as angina pectoris, left ventricular failure, pulmonary thromboembolism, and ventricular arrhythmias. [3]

4.4.3. Diagnosis

The electrocardiogram may show persistence ST segment elevation. Echocardiography can visualize the aneurysm and also, evaluate the presence of intracavitary thrombus. Coronary angiography and hemodynamic studies are indicated for the diagnosis and may guide the surgical procedure. [2]

4.4.4. Surgical treatment

Surgical treatment should be performed only after the healing phase of AMI, which lasts about six weeks, because of the friable tissues surrounding the infarcted area, raising surgical risks. However, it must be urgently done in cases of cardiogenic shock refractory to medical therapy, or in the presence of ventricular arrhythmias, refractory to conventional treatment. [2, 3]

From the hemodynamic point of view, the goals

The main objectives to be achieved with the surgical treatment are to increased ejection fraction, reduce the final diastolic volume and carry out an appropriate coronary graft bypass. [1]

The current mortality rates in the surgical treatment ranges from 3.3 to 7.2%, but in patients with severe ventricular dysfunction it may reach 19%. Patients with successful surgical treatment have a significant improvement in their functional class and have a 5-year survival of 60%. [2, 3]

The sequence for the treatment of ventricular aneurysm is based on: [1, 18]

1. Definition of the aneurysm;
2. Careful intracavitary thrombus removal;
3. Recognition of the area to be resected;
4. Elimination of the septum´s paradoxical pulse area;
5. Reconstruction of the ventricle, with or without prosthetic tissue as a patch.

The techniques for surgical correction of this complication include: [1, 2, 7]

- Resection of the aneurysmal area of the left ventricle, with linear suture of the edges;
- Replacement of the ventricular wall by prosthetic material (Dacron);
- Reconstruction of left ventricular geometry, using Dacron or bovine pericardium ;
- Endoaneurysmorrhaphy use of synthetic material sutured inside the ventricular cavity;

- Endoaneurysmorrhaphy using semi-rigid prosthesis of bovine pericardium;
- Ablation of ventricular arrhythmia foci, usually in fibrous areas of the myocardium, identified by intraoperative electrophysiological mapping.

5. Mechanical complications of acute myocardial infarction — Results

The main surgical considerations: [7]

a. preoperative coronary angiography to investigate lesions in other coronary arteries also need intervention when possible;

b. early intervention to reduce infarct size and rapidly reperfuse the ischemic myocardium;

c. femoral cannulation to prevent exsanguination in cases of rupture of the ventricular free wall;

d. use of mechanical circulatory support devices such as intra-aortic balloon (IAB) to increase coronary perfusion pressure and reduce afterload;

e. approaching the area without viability of the left ventricle, with repair of the interventricular septum followed by infarctectomy;

f. myocardial revascularization procedure in the same act, whenever possible, to improve long-term prognosis.

The main determinants of increased mortality are: preoperative hemodynamic instability, the presence of multiple organ failure, and the need for concomitant CABG surgery along with the correction of the defect.

Mortality in clinical and surgical treatment of mechanical complications of acute myocardial infarction can be seen in table 5:

	Ventricularfreewallrupture	Ventricular Septum Rupture	IschemicPapillaryMuscle Rupture	Left Ventrícular Aneurysm
Clinical treatment	About 100%	About 94%	About 71%	about 49%, 80% within the first 5 days post AMI
Surgical treatment	About 60%	20 - 60%; 87% in cardiogenic shock	4-13% (mild); 30-70% (severe); medium 20% (30-40% within 5 years)	3,3 - 7,2%, rising to 19% in cardiogenic shock (40% within 5 years)

Table 5. Mortality rates of patients from mechanical complications of acute myocardial infarction [2, 3, 14, 15, 16]

http://dx.doi.org/10.5772/57110

6. Conclusion

Patients with mechanical complications of acute myocardial infarction (ventricular free wall rupture, ventricular septal rupture and mitral regurgitation with hemodynamic, pulmonary congestion and / or cardiogenic shock) should undergo emergency surgery, according to the guidelines of the American Heart Association (Class I, level of evidence B). The coronary artery bypass surgery, whenever possible, should be performed during surgery.

Author details

Luís Augusto Palma Dallan, Luiz Roberto Palma Dallan, Luiz Augusto Ferreira Lisboa and Luís Alberto Oliveira Dallan

Heart Institute, University of São Paulo Medical School, Brazil

References

[1] Dallan LAO, Lisboa LAF, Almeida SA. Complicações Mecânicas do Infarto Agudo do Miocárdio. In: Porto CC – Doenças do Coração: Prevenção e Terapêutica. Ed Guanabara-Koogan, 2 ed, Rio de Janeiro 2005; pp 691 – 709.

[2] III Direttriz sobre o tratamento do infarto agudo do miocárdio – Sociedade Brasileira de Cardiologia. Arq Bras Cardiol 2004; 83

[3] Antman EM, Ambe DT, Armstrong PW et al. – ACC / AHA guidelines for the management of patients with ST-Elevation myocardial infarction: a report of the American College of Cardiology / American Heart Association Task Force on practice guidelines 2004.

[4] Jatene FB, Monteiro R, Hueb AC. Intervenções Cirúrgicas na Doença Arterial Coronária Aguda. In Nobre F, Serrano Jr CV (eds): Tratado de Cardiologia SOCESP. 1 ed. São Paulo, ed. Manole 2005, p. 719-727.

[5] Nicolau JC e Marin-Neto JA (eds)– Síndromes isquêmicas miocárdicas instáveis. São Paulo, ed. Atheneu, 2001,

[6] Abreu Filho CAC, Dallan LAO, Lisboa LAF et al. Tratamento cirúrgico da rotura da parede livre do ventrículo esquerdo após infarto agudo do miocárdio. Rev Bras Cir Cardiovasc 2002; 17:6-13.

[7] Massad MG, Geha, AS. Surgical repair of mechanical complications of myocardial infarction. World J Surg 2004; 28:847-856

[8] Buda AJ. The role of echocardiography in the evaluation of mechanical complications of acute myocardial infarction. Circulation 1991; 84:109-121.

[9] Reddy SG, Roberts WC. Frequency of rupture of the left ventricular free wall or ventricular septum among necropsy cases of fatal acute myocardial infarction since introduction of coronary care unit. Am J Cardiol 1989; 63:906-11

[10] Lima RC, Kubrusly LF; Nery AC et al. Diretrizes da cirurgia de revascularização miocárdica. Sociedade Brasileira de Cardiologia. Arq Bras Cardiol 2004; 82:1-20.

[11] Braunwald E. Heart disease a textbook of cardiovascular medicine. 5th ed, Philadelphia, WB Saunders, 1997.

[12] Dallan LAO, Oliveira SA, Abreu Fo CA et al. Infarto hemorrágico conseqüente à reperfusão miocárdica. Relato de quatro casos. Arq Bras Cardiol, 1990; 54:127-132.

[13] Dallan LAO, Oliveira SA, Abreu Fo CA et al. Rotura cardíaca após infarto agudo do miocárdio: uma complicação passível de correção cirúrgica? Rev Bras Cir Cardiovasc 1993; 8[4]:272-281.

[14] Dallan LAO, Oliveira SA, Atik F et al. Insuficiência valvar mitral isquêmica. Incidência, diagnóstico e tratamento cirúrgico. Arq Bras Cardiol, 1994; 62:329-336

[15] The GUSTO investigators. An international randomized trial comparing four thrombolitic strategies for acute myocardial infarction. N Engl J Med 1993; 329:673-82

[16] Sanborn TA, Bates ER, Jacobs AK et al. Impact of thrombolysis, intra-aortic balloon pump counter-pulsation, and their combination in cardiogenic shock complicating acute myocaldial infarction: a report from the SHOCK trial registry. Should we emergently revascularize occluded coronaries for cardiogenic shock? J Am Coll Cardiol 2000; 36: 1123-9

[17] Gutierrez PS, Higushi MI, Moraes CF et al. Diferentas entre homens e mulheres em casos fatais de infarto do miocárdio: estudo de duzentas necropsias. Arq Bras Cardiol 1990; 54:189-92.

[18] Jatene AD. Ventricular Aneurismectomy. Ressection or reconstruction. Torac Cardiovasc Surg 1985; 89[3]:321. ISIS-2 (Second International Study of Infarct Survival) Collaborative Group. Randomised trial of intravenous streptokinase, oral aspirin, both, or neither among 17,187 cases of suspected acute myocardial infarction: ISIS-2. Lancet 1988; ii: 349-360.

Chapter 8

Hypoplastic Left Heart Syndrome: Why Use a Hybrid Procedure?

Miguel Maluf

Additional information is available at the end of the chapter

http://dx.doi.org/10.5772/57116

1. Introduction

Neonates with hypoplastic left heart syndrome (HLHS) and its variants have diminutive left-sided structures with systemic outflow obstruction and subsequent duct-dependent systemic, cerebral, and coronary circulations. [1]

Bilateral PA banding was described by Norwood based on his early experience of surgical palliation for HLHS before he established the 'Norwood procedure [2] and has been an option to stabilize critically ill neonates with HLHS.[3] This procedure, however, did not become a hybrid procedure until ductal stenting became clinically available.

The Norwood procedure has been the sole option to achieve these purposes for nearly 20 years. [4], [5] Despite a significant improvement in survival after stage I palliation, early mortality remains as high as 20-30% [6], [7] with significant morbidity, including neurologic injury. [8], [9], due to deep hypothermia, cardiocirculatory arrest, prolonged cardiopulmonary bypass, sternum delayed closure, use of extracorporeal membrane oxygenator (ECMO) and prolonged Hospital stay.

Survivors Norwood op. are showing suboptimal neurological development. (Figure 1)

In the last decade the hybrid procedure has emerged as an alternative stage I palliation in neonates with HLHS. (Gibbs et al) [10].: Stenting of the arterial duct combined with banding of the pulmonary arteries and atrial septectomy or septostomy: a new approach to palliation for the hypoplastic left heart syndrome

This review discusses the historical aspect, surgical and interventional techniques, current outcomes and future direction of this procedure.(Figure 2)

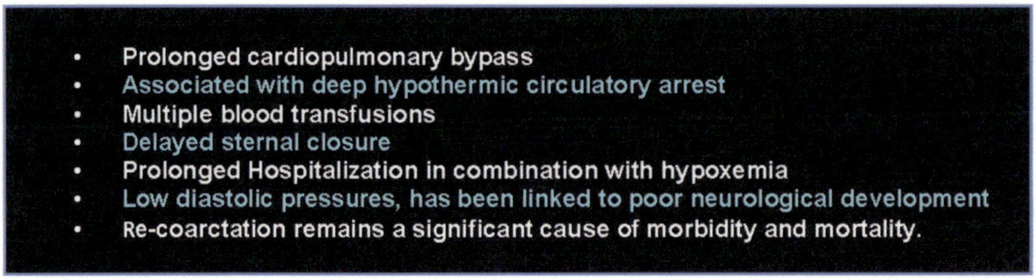

Figure 1. Causes of suboptimal neurologic development

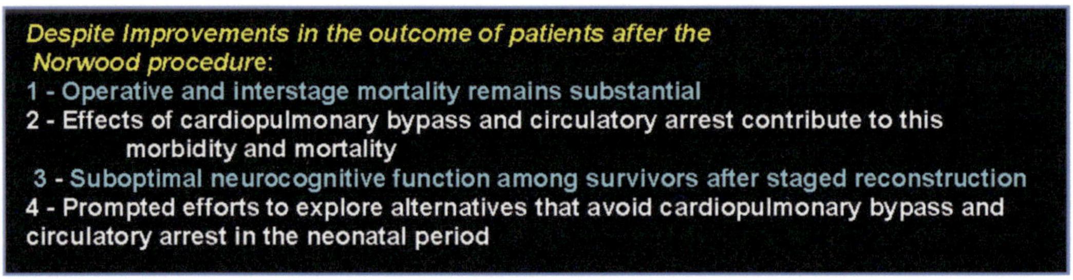

Figure 2. Vantages of Hybrid Procedures in patients with Hypoplastic Left Heart Syndrome

Hybrid palliation yields equivalent but not superior stage I palliation survival and comparable 1-year survival to conventional Norwood palliation, comparable pre-stage II hemodynamics and pulmonary artery growth, and preserved ventricular function in stage II palliation. Hybrid palliation utilizes significantly less resource and shortens postoperative recovery. In comprehensive stage II palliation the impact of pulmonary artery reconstruction on subsequent pulmonary artery growth has not been determined and should be further investigated. A prospective, randomized trial is warranted to compare these two surgical strategies for neonates with hypoplastic left heart syndrome.

The high mortality and morbidity stems from the following two components: an essentially unstable "in-parallel" circulation of Norwood physiology with a systemic-to-pulmonary shunt, and surgical stress driven by cardiopulmonary bypass (CPB), deep hypothermic circulatory arrest (DHCA), and the subsequent systemic inflammatory response.

2. Hybrid procedure

2.1. Indications

In High-risk patients:

- Aortic atresia

- Severe non-cardiac anomalies
- Low body weight (<2.5 kg)
- Intact or highly restrictive atrial septum
- Prematurity
- Poor ventricular function
- Diminutive aortic arch
- Stenotic aortic isthmus

The HLHS variants, such as tricuspid atresia with transposed great arteries, unbalanced atrioventricular septal defect with aortic arch obstruction, or double inlet left ventricle with transposed great arteries, are all considered an indication for the hybrid procedure. [11]

Staged surgical palliation with the standard Norwood approach, hybrid approach, and primary transplantation are equally offered to the patient's family by the cardiologist, and no specific decision-making protocol is applied

In patients with aortic atresia, the coronary and cerebral circulations are entirely dependent on retrograde blood flow through the aortic isthmus. If there are any signs of pre-operative obstruction at the aortic isthmus or retrograde aortic arch, deployment of a ductal stent can result in acute or chronic obstruction of the aortic isthmus, leading to coronary and cerebral ischemia.[12] This specific anatomic feature can be a relative contraindication for a 'conventional' hybrid procedure [13] unless specific measures are applied to secure the coronary and cerebral circulations:

Surgical procedures proposes

- Prophylactic main PA to innominate artery shunt during stage I palliation: Reverse Blalock-Taussig (BT) shunt
- Stent placement in the stenotic aortic isthmus
- Avoidance of the hybrid procedure in favor of the Norwood procedure or transplantation.
- Operative Techniques
- Hybrid procedure for the treatment of HLHS is preferably indicated in the following situations (Figure 3)

2.2. Stage I palliation

2.2.1. Hybrid stage I

The first hybrid procedure for the palliative treatment of HLHS,was held in São Paulo Federal University, was held in 1995 in a patient 30 days, weight 3,800 grams by reason of the refusal of parents to the procedures offered: Op Norwood or heart transplant [14]

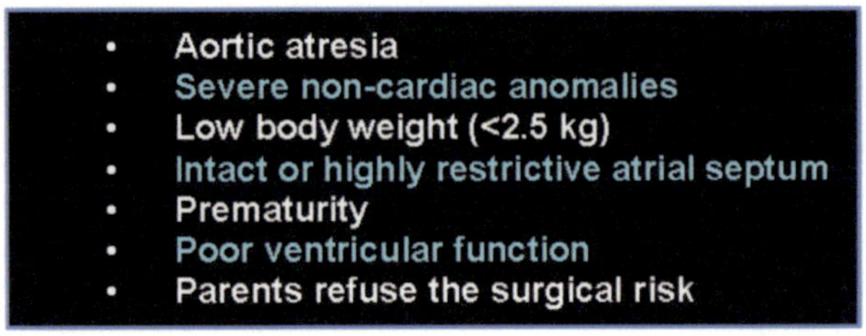

Figure 3. Indication Hybrid procedure

Palliation has been previously described. [9, 10] Herein, the current techniques used in The Hospital for Sick Children are described. The procedure is performed in the catheterization laboratory, which is referred to as the 'hybrid suite'. Under general anesthesia, a median sternotomy is made and the thymus is resected. Bilateral PA banding is achieved using a 3.5 mm polytetrafluoroethylene graft, which is divided longitudinally and wrapped around the branch PAs for a width of approximately 3 mm.

The bands are then secured to the adventitia of the main PA with 5-0 or 6-0 non-absorbable polypropylene sutures to avoid distal dislodging. A vascular clip is placed at the proximal edge of the left PA band to guide the interventionist for ductal stenting.

The patient is partially heparinized, a purse-string suture is placed on the main PA, and a 6-Fr sheath is inserted. The ductal stent is deployed through the sheath under fluoroscopic guidance, achieving stage I palliation (Figs. 4, 5, 6, 7 and 8). We currently use a self-expanding stent, 20 mm in length and 8-10 mm in diameter

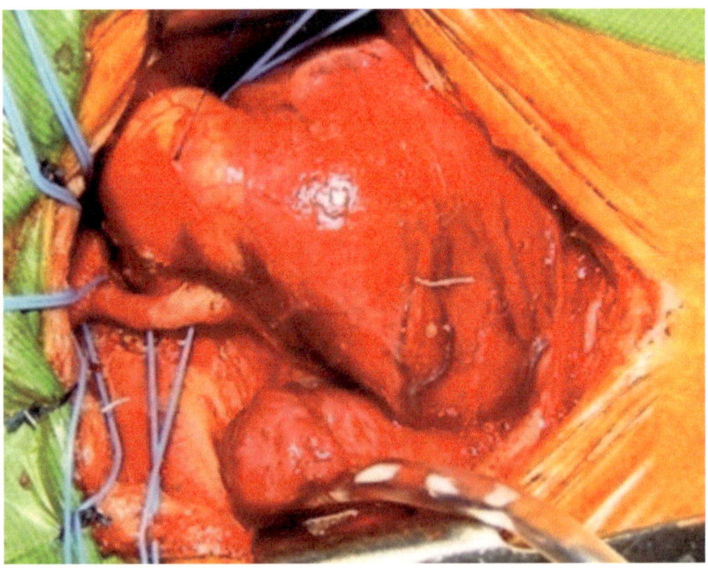

Figure 4. Surgical view – Case with Hypoplastic Left Heart Syndrome (HLHS)

http://dx.doi.org/10.5772/57116

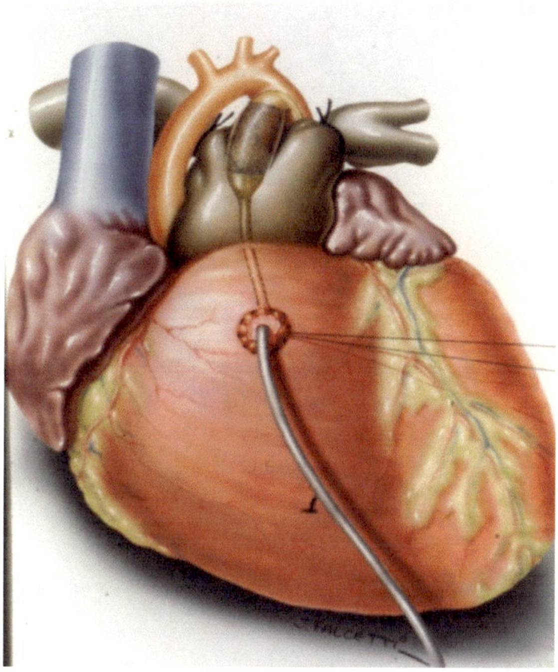

Figure 5. Surgical draw of hybrid procedure: A purse-string suture is placed on the main PA, and a 6-Fr sheath is inserted. The ductal stent is deployed through the sheath under fluoroscopic guidance, achieving stage I palliation

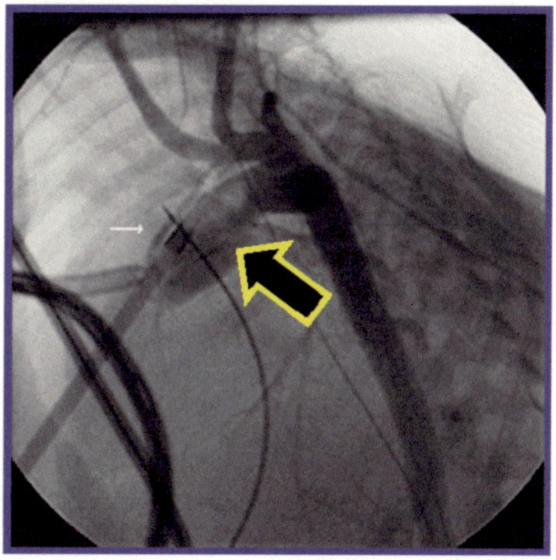

Figure 6. Angiographic study during stent deployment in hybrid stage I palliation. The lateral view showing the sheath and guide wire inserted via the main PA through the Arterial Duct. (arrow)

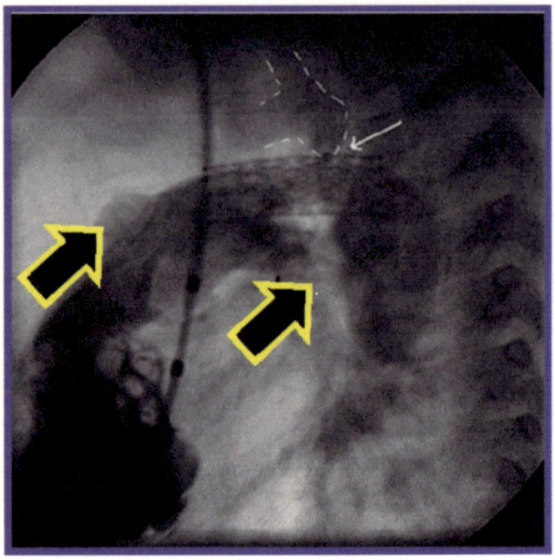

Figure 7. Angiographic sequence of stent deployment in hybrid stage I palliation. The lateral view showing the stent into arterial duct (thin arrow) and bilateral banding of the Pas (large arrow).

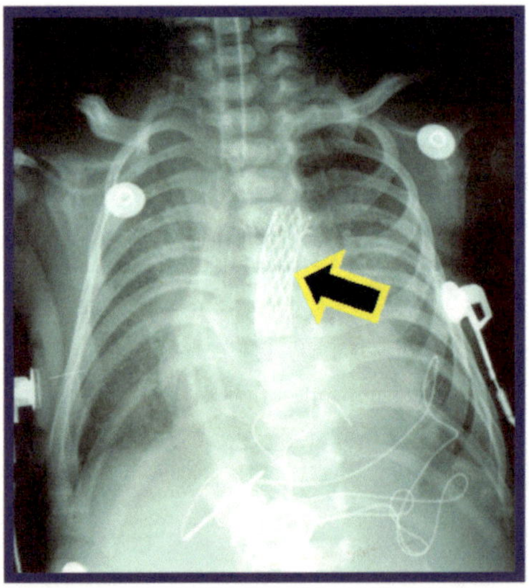

Figure 8. Post-operative Chest X Ray showing the stent into the Arterial Duct (arrow)

- Milrinone is commonly used in post-operative care to optimize cardiac output and provide systemic vasodilatation. This management strategy stems from our early observation that patients who underwent a hybrid procedure had diminished cardiac output, high systemic vascular resistance, and a high pulmonary-to-systemic flow ratio (Qp/Qs) despite avoiding CPB/DHCA.

- In our early experience, atrial septectomy was typically performed as part of the same procedure; currently atrial septectomy and stenting are deferred until the intra-atrial communication becomes restrictive.

Reverse Blalock-Taussig shunt

- In patients with aortic atresia or those thought to have severely restricted prograde aortic flow, a revered BT shunt is prophylactically placed from the main PA to the innominate artery.. After bilateral PA banding is achieved, a side-biting clamp is placed on the main PA and proximal anastomosis is made using a 3.5 or 4 mm polytetrafluoroethylene graft on the anterior wall of the main PA. Distal anastomosis is then performed to the proximal innominate artery with a standard anastomotic technique. [11].The flow in the shunt is directed from the main PA to the innominate artery. Ductal stenting is then performed.

Interstage monitoring

- Close monitoring with weekly or biweekly clinic visits and echocardiograms are performed. The arm-leg blood pressure difference is measured at every clinic visit to exclude any signs of aortic arch obstruction. Echocardiographic follow-up is particularly focused on the presence or absence of flow acceleration in the aortic isthmus, indicating progression of retrograde aortic arch obstruction. The status of the atrial septum is also carefully monitored, determining the timing of atrial septectomy. There are no certain criteria for intervention on the atrial septum. The decision is made based on the balance between the patient's clinical status and the pressure gradient across the intra-atrial communication. A mild-to-moderate pressure gradient up to 8-10 mmHg is acceptable as long as the patient is thriving. Prompt intervention is required when the patient has symptoms of left atrial hypertension, such as poor feeding, an increased respiratory rate, and a decrease in arterial saturation.

- Ventricular function and atrioventricular valve regurgitation are of great importance during the follow-up echocardiographic examination. Depressed ventricular function can be a result of retrograde aortic arch obstruction in the setting of minimal or no antegrade aortic flow, or stenosis of a reverse BT shunt. The patency and flow pattern of the reverse BT shunt is documented. Anti-platelet and/or anti-coagulation is indicated only if the patient has a reverse BT shunt. Anti-platelet therapy is initiated if the patient has a stent across the atrial septum. Pre-stage II cardiac catheterization is electively performed at 3-4 months of age unless intervention for the atrial septum is necessary at an earlier age.

3. Conclusion

- Thus, it remains of outmost importance to determine the outcome of children treated with hybrid procedure in comparison to that of the Norwood procedure to establish the best treatment strategy for this most vulnerable population.

- This can only be achieved by performing a large multicenter randomized trial, in which the effect size can be based on the results of our study and in which all potential risk factors such as preoperative delayed brain development and brain injury, intra- and postoperative factors and socio-demographic factors need to be considered.

Author details

Miguel Maluf*

Associate Professor - Cardiovascular Division, Universidade Federal de São Paulo, Brazil

References

[1] Noonan JA, Nadas AS. The hypoplastic left heart syndrome: an analysis of 101 cases. Pediatr Clin North Am. 1958;5:1029–1056.

[2] Lang P, Norwood WI. Hemodynamic assessment after palliative surgery for hypoplastic left heart syndrome. Circulation. 1983;68:104–108.

[3] Pizarro C, Norwood WI. Pulmonary artery banding before Norwood procedure. Ann Thorac Surg. 2003;75:1008–1010.

[4] Norwood WI, Lang P, Hansen DD. Physiologic repair of aortic atresia-hypoplastic left heart syndrome. N Engl J Med. 1983;308:23–26.

[5] Mahle WT, Spray TL, Wernovsky G, Gaynor JW, Clark BJ., 3rd Survival after reconstructive surgery for hypoplastic left heart syndrome: a 15-year experience from a single institution. Circulation. 2000;102(19 Suppl 3):

[6] De Oliveira NC, Ashburn DA, Khalid F, et al. Prevention of early sudden circulatory collapse after the Norwood operation. Circulation. 2004;110(11 Suppl 1)

[7] Stasik CN, Gelehrter S, Goldberg CS, Bove EL, Devaney EJ, Ohye RG. Current outcomes and risk factors for the Norwood procedure. J Thorac Cardiovasc Surg. 2006;131:412–417.

[8] Goldberg CS, Schwartz EM, Brunberg JA, et al. Neurodevelopmental outcome of patients after the fontan operation: a comparison between children with hypoplastic left heart syndrome and other functional single ventricle lesions. J Pediatr. 2000;137:646–652.

[9] Galli KK, Zimmerman RA, Jarvik GP, et al. Periventricular leukomalacia is common after neonatal cardiac surgery. J Thorac Cardiovasc Surg. 2004;127:692–704.

[10] Gibbs JL, Wren C, Watterson KG, Hunter S, Hamilton JR. Stenting of the arterial duct combined with banding of the pulmonary arteries and atrial septectomy or septosto-

http://dx.doi.org/10.5772/57116

my: a new approach to palliation for the hypoplastic left heart syndrome. Br Heart J 1993;69:551-555

[11] 11-Osami Honjo, Christopher A. Caldarone. Hybrid Palliation for Neonates With Hypoplastic Left Heart Syndrome: Current Strategies and Outcomes. Korean Circ J. 2010 March; 40(3): 103–111.

[12] Caldarone CA, Benson LN, Holtby H, Van Arsdell GS. Main pulmonary artery to innominate artery shunt during hybrid palliation of hypoplastic left heart syndrome. J Thorac Cardiovasc Surg. 2005;130:

[13] Stoica S, Philips A, Egan M, et al. The Retrograde Aortic Arch in the Hybrid Approach to Hypoplastic Left Heart Syndrome Society for Thoracic Surgeons 45th Annual Meeting; San Fransicsio. 2009.

[14] Maluf M A Pediatric Cardiac Surgery: A challenge of skill and creativity in constant search results. Book: Contemporary Pediatrics – Ed.: ntech, March 2012, Chapter 9, pg.: 201-280.

Chapter 9

Surgical Repair of Stenotic Pulmonary Arteries in Tetralogy of Falllot

Vinicius José da Silva Nina

Additional information is available at the end of the chapter

http://dx.doi.org/10.5772/57111

1. Introduction

Tetralogy of Fallot (TOF), primarily named La Maladie Bleue by Louis Arthur Etienne Fallot in 1888, is the clinical description of the physiology created by a combination of anatomic malformations that consists of an interventricular communication, or ventricular septal defect, biventricular connection of the aortic root, which overrides the muscular ventricular septum, obstruction of the right ventricular outflow tract, and right ventricular hypertrophy. This cyanotic malformation belongs to a family of diseases characterized by a similar intracardiac anatomy but highly variable in terms of pulmonary artery anatomy, associated abnormalities, and outcomes; once each component can vary in its severity, with the variation directly affecting the manifestation and management of the disease.

Although the stenosis of the pulmonary trunk and its bifurcation is uncommon, the right and left pulmonary arteries are stenotic to some degree in 30% of infants with Tetralogy of Fallot presenting in the first year of life [1-3].

Based on this premise, here we focus on pulmonary artery anatomy which is one of the most challenging components of Tetralogy of Fallot especially regarding the complexity of its surgical repair and the selection of materials to accomplish such repair. Decision making, timing and techniques for repairing each of these pulmonary artery variants are emphasized in this chapter according to the authors experience and also based on the best evidence in the literature.

2. Morphologic categories of pulmonary artery anatomy in Tetralogy of Fallot

Size and configuration of the pulmonary arteries have been thought to be important determinants of postoperative right ventricular function after complete repair of tetralogy of Fallot. As such, they may affect the result of repair when the pulmonary arteries are hypoplastic or stenotic [1].

Hypoplasia or narrowness, in the arterial pathways in patients having TOF with pulmonary stenosis is most marked centrally in the RV infundibulum and pulmonary trunk. On average, the RPA and LPA and their branches are not abnormally small. This does not deny the occasional existence of severe narrowing at the origin of the LPA or RPA. Elzenga et al [5] found juxtaductal proximal stenosis of the LPA in 10% of patients having TOF with pulmonary stenosis; about 90% are free of these severe finding [4, 6].

The nearly infinitely variable spectrum of pulmonary artery obstruction in TOF can be conveniently categorized in a way that is surgically useful because it relates to difficulty in obtaining good relief of the pulmonary stenosis and therefore to surgical techniques and mortality. Because of this great variability in the dimensions of the pulmonary arteries, their careful pre-repair study is very important. In this regard we have didactically separated the pulmonary artery tree into three anatomical segments:

- pulmonary trunk;
- pulmonary trunk bifurcation and;
- pulmonary branches (right and left pulmonary arteries).

3. Pulmonary trunk

In TOF, the pulmonary trunk is nearly always smaller than the aorta. Reduction is most marked when there is a diffuse RV outflow hypoplasia. In this case, the pulmonary trunk is less than half the aortic diameter and is short, directed sharply posterior to its bifurcation. It is largely hidden from view at operation by the prominent aorta, which also displaces the origin of the trunk leftward and posteriorly [4].

When the pulmonary valve is markedly dysplastic, the pulmonary trunk is also stenotic or corseted at its commissural attachments, and it may be very angulated or kinked at this point. This is the usual mechanism of supravalvar narrowing, and it is not associated with wall thickening. Rarely, however, there may be a discrete supravalvar narrowing beyond commissural level with diffuse wall thickening [1, 6].

4. Pulmonary trunk bifurcation

The left pulmonary artery (LPA) is usually a direct continuation of the pulmonary trunk; with the right pulmonary artery (RPA) arising almost at right angles and close to it, but this pattern varies. In TOF is uncommon to have the distal pulmonary trunk and origin of RPA and LPA being moderately or severely narrowed (bifurcation stenosis), and in this situation the bifurcation may have a Y shape [7] (Fig.1)

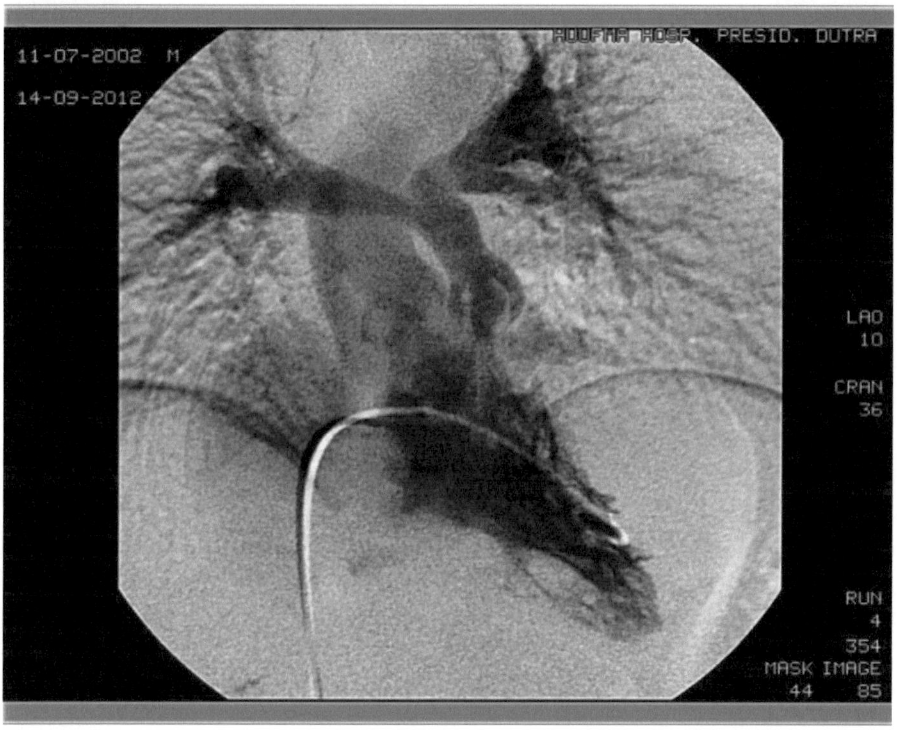

Figure 1. Angiogram showing stenosis of distal pulmonary trunk. Note that the LPA is a continuation of the pulmonary trunk.

5. Right and left pulmonary arteries

Although anomalies of the RPA and LPA are more common in TOF with pulmonary atresia rather than stenosis, Fellows et al found pulmonary artery anomalies in 30% of infants having TOF with pulmonary stenosis presenting in the first year of life [4,8].

The more severe the hypoplasia of the infundibulum and pulmonary trunk, the more severe is the narrowing of the first part of the right and left pulmonary arteries, although the Z values of these structures are usually larger than those of the pulmonary trunk [6]. (Fig.2)

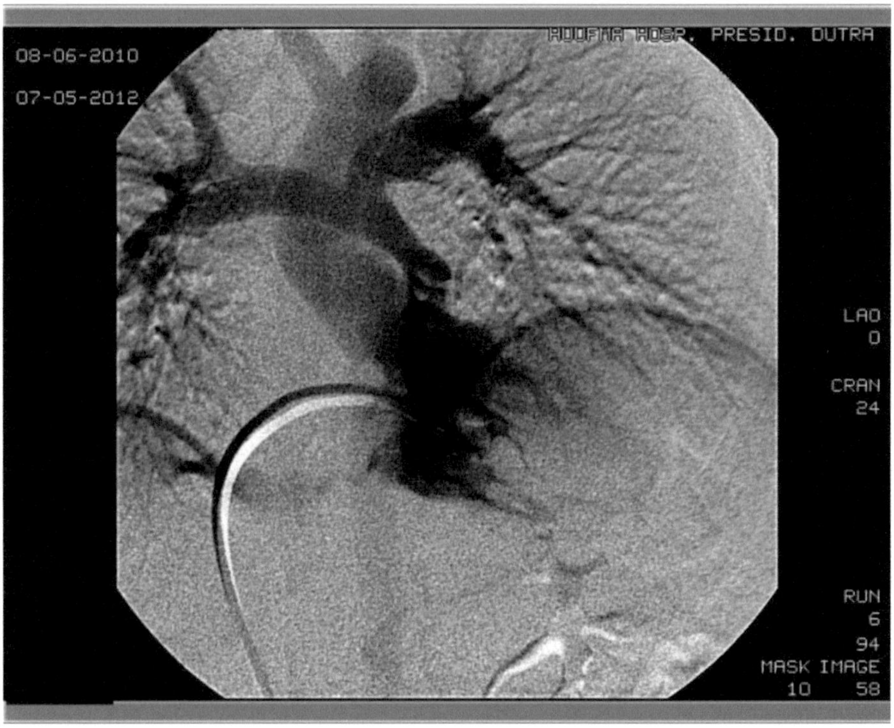

Figure 2. Angiogram showing stenosis of pulmonary trunk bifurcation. Note the Y shape of the pulmonary trunk bifurcation.

6. Surgical approach over the pulmonary trunk and branches

Pulmonary artery branch stenoses are widely known congenital anomalies especially in children with TOF. Many authors have reported hypoplastic or stenotic pulmonary artery branches to be a major obstacle to successful operative correction of TOF [7,9-13].

In this section we present different techniques and materials that can be used to repair such diseased pulmonary arteries according to their location, size and anatomical configuration.

7. Pulmonary trunk stenosis

In cases of pulmonary trunk stenosis some steps must be followed in order to obtain a successful surgical repair:

1. Sizing the pulmonary trunk

If the pulmonary valve annulus is hypoplastic, the infundibulotomy incision is extended across the annulus between the valve commissures as far as needed (up to the bifurcation or up to the left or right pulmonary artery). The size of the pulmonary trunk and of the left and right pulmonary arteries is measured by Hegar probes, and then those arteries are calibrated to fit a normal diameter, adjusted to the child's body surface area [14-16].(Table 1)

BSA (m^2)	Pulmonary Annulus
0.25	8.4
0.30	9.3
0.35	10.1
0.40	10.7
0.45	11.3
0.50	11.9
0.60	12.8
0.70	13.5
0.80	14.2
0.90	14.8
1.0	15.3
1.2	16.2
1.4	17.0
1.6	17.6
1.8	18.2
2.0	19.0
Data from Rowlatt et at. [14]	

Table 1. Mean normal diameter of pulmonary valve

In some patients the distal pulmonary trunk is narrower than the annulus; in these cases the incision is extended into the LPA, which usually continues in the same general direction as the pulmonary trunk and is usually proportionally larger than the distal pulmonary trunk. If the origin of the LPA is proportionally no larger than the distal pulmonary trunk, then the incision and patch reconstruction should be carried into the mid portion of the LPA, which is nearly always wider than the origin [1,4,6].

2. Measuring the patch

Generally, a transannular patch should not be placed when the Z value is larger than -3. Otherwise, the incision is carried across the annulus, the pulmonary valve excised, and the patch inserted.

The length of the patch can be determined by measuring length of the incision from the RV to the pulmonary artery, and its maximum width is determined visually by holding the edges of the incision open at valve level and judging the size of the roof required to create a new pulmonary annulus whose diameter is no larger than three fourths the diameter of the ascending aorta [4,17] (Fig. 3).

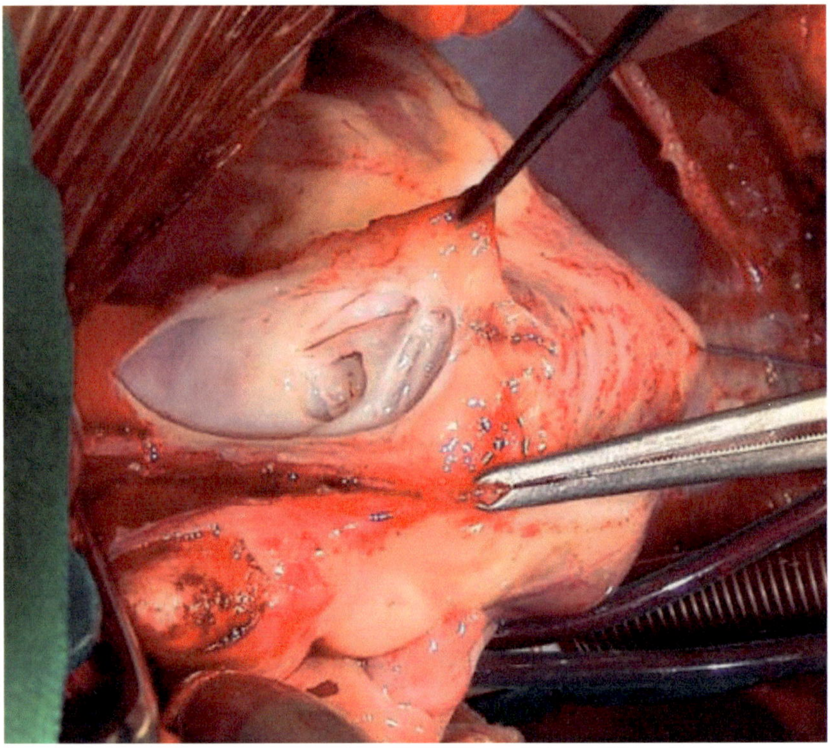

Figure 3. Measuring the patch. Pulmonary trunk opened with a dysplastic pulmonary valve (From Jacob M F F B et al [17] with permission)

Alternatively a Hegar dilator can be placed through the divided annulus and the width of the patch required to complete the roof over it measured. Usually, the patch is about 50mm long and 15mm wide at its center. Both ends are cut almost transversely to create a blunt patch. When a transannular patch is used, a major consideration is the distal extent of the incision in the pulmonary trunk, because this must be into an area of distinctly greater diameter than that of the annulus, which is usually the narrowest area [4,17] (Fig. 4)

3. Selecting the patch

The transannular patch may be of glutaraldehyde-treated or untreated pericardium. Glutaraldehyde-treated pericardium is advantageous because it facilitates precise sizing of the patch, and when properly trimmed, its convexity is ensured, as is a relatively square cut of its distal end. Thus, when it is inserted, it forms a roof that is convex in all directions relieving the transpulmonary gradient. Although technically more demanding; untreated, especially pedicled pericardium has the potential advantage of growing as the child grows [9,10,17,18].

http://dx.doi.org/10.5772/57111

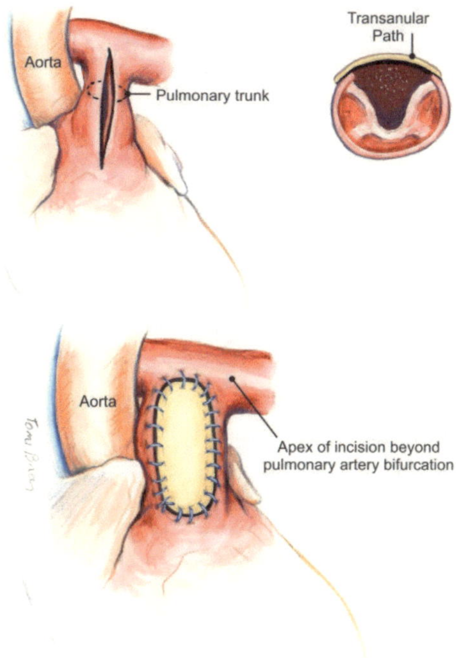

Figure 4. Transannular patch repair of TOF with pulmonary stenosis. Note the pericardial roofing to enlarge the valve annulus and proximal pulmonary trunk..

4. Inserting the patch

a. Glutaraldehyde-treated pericardium

The patch is positioned using continuous 5-0 polypropylene sutures, commencing at the distal end of the incision. The suture is mattressed at the end and over and over elsewhere, placing the first two or three throws along each side before pulling the pericardial patch into position as the suture is tightened. Suturing is continued down each side to annulus level; then the reminder of the right ventriculotomy is closed by incorporating the pericardial patch into it with continuous sutures. Deep bites of muscle are taken down each side and at the angle [17] (Fig 5).

b. Untratead pedicled pericardium

- Preparation and tailoring of the pericardial flap:

The broadly based pericardial flaps are tailored before cardiopulmonary bypass begins. The pericardial sac is usually opened transversely in the midline near the diaphragm. The incision is extended along the diaphragm toward both phrenic nerves and then goes cephalad, parallelling the right phrenic nerve closely, until the flap can be rotated in front of the pulmonary arterial segment needed to be repaired. The pericardium usually remained normally attached on the left side with the left phrenic nerve along its base [18,19] (Fig. 6).

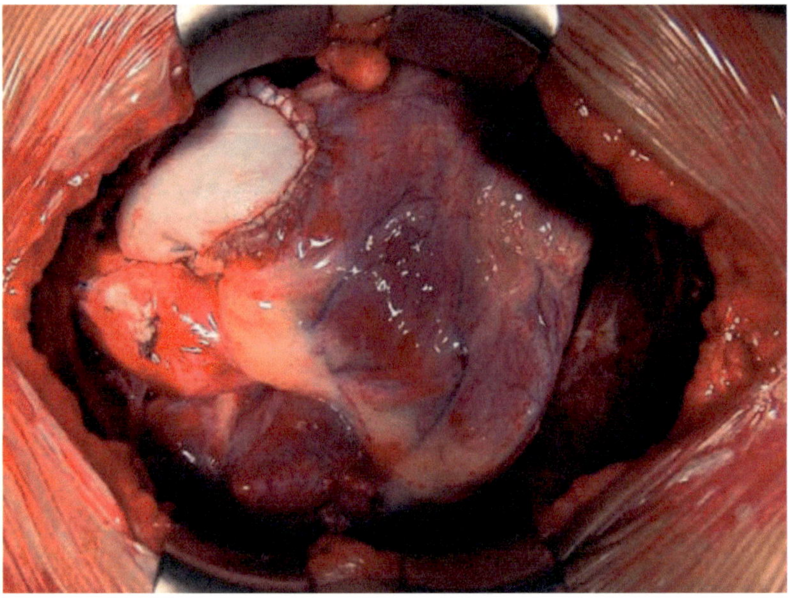

Figure 5. Enlargement of the right ventricular outflow tract with bovine pericardium patch. (From Jacob M F F B et al [17] with permission)

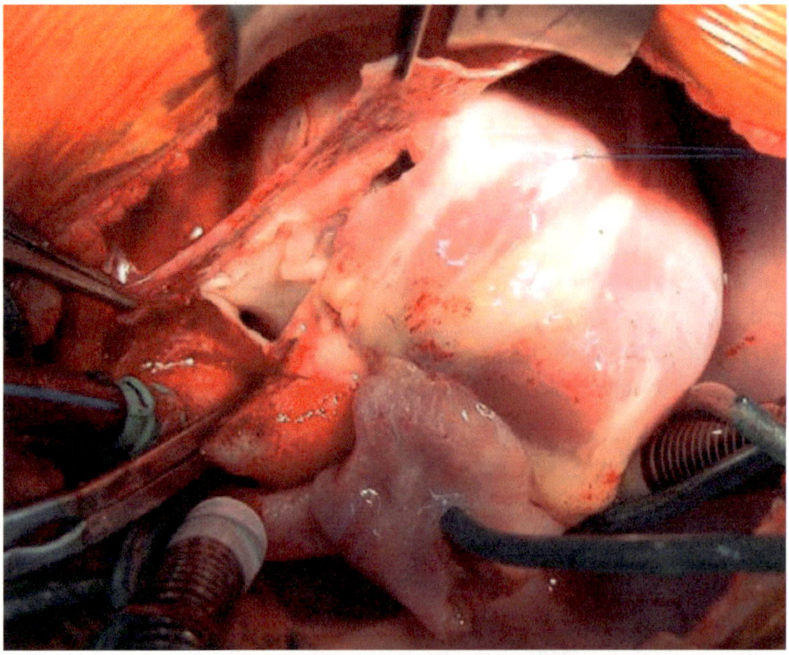

Figure 6. Surgical aspect of the pedicled autologous pericardium (tweezers) before enlargement. The anterior side of the right ventricular outflow tract, valve ring and pulmonary trunk can also be observed. (From Croti, UA et al [18] with permission)

http://dx.doi.org/10.5772/57111

• Inserting the pedicled pericardium patch

After incising the anterior aspect of the pulmonary trunk, pulmonary valve ring and right ventricular outflow tract, the valve ring is measured using Hegar dilator according to the body surface area as previously described, then the suture of the pericardium is begun at the lateral edge by implanting the patch on a tile-shaped using 6-0 polydioxanone thread throughout the suture.

The aim of this approach is to allow for growth and to avoid future calcification, among other known problems existing with several materials that can be used for this purpose [19] (Fig.7).

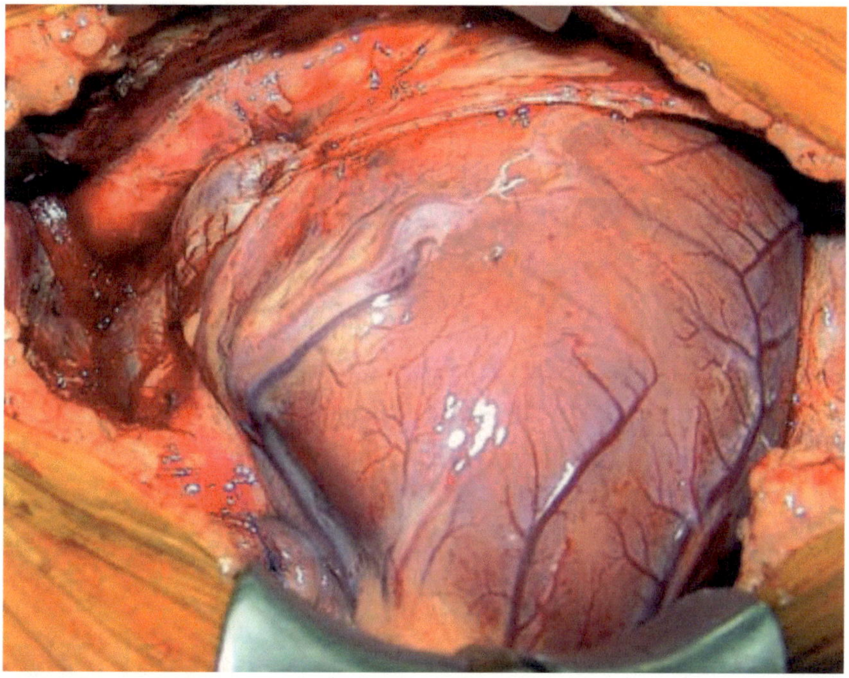

Figure 7. Final aspect after pedicled autologous pericardium implantation to enlarge the right ventricular outflow tract, valve ring and pulmonary trunk (From Croti, UA et al [18] with permission)

• Using a valved patch

If it is anticipated that a too large transannular patch will be required, a monocusp may be attached to the pericardial roofing patch to prevent increasing postoperative pulmonary regurgitation. The cusp diameter is fashioned somewhat larger than the planned roofed RV outflow. It is cut more or less circular and sutured to the patch when the latter suturing from distally reaches the valve annulus. Numerous materials, such as polytetrafluoroethylene, porcine heterografts, allografts and others can also be used to repair the pulmonary trunk in this situation [21,22](Fig.8).

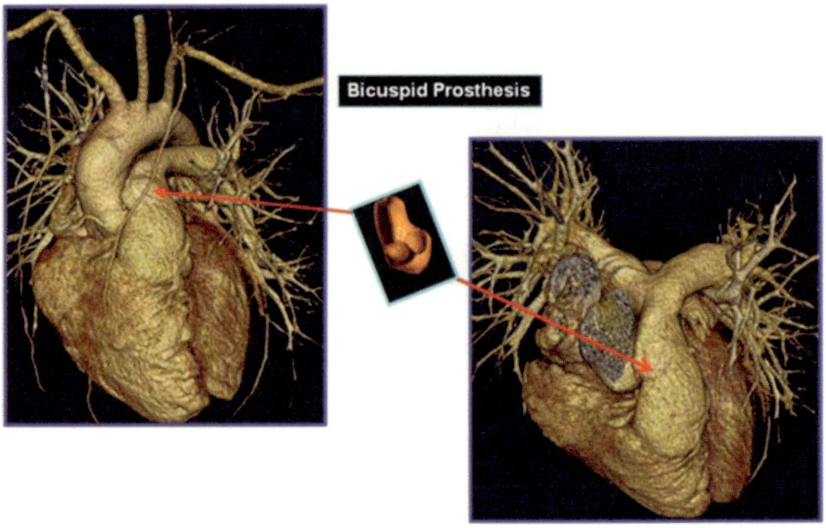

Figure 8. Computerized tomography in a patient with tetralogy of Fallot submitted to surgical repair of the right ventricular outflow tract with an implant of a preserved porcine pulmonary bicuspid prosthesis (inset). (From Maluf MA et al [21] with permission)

If the surgeon's preference is for a monocusp allograft and, considering that only one cusp will be used and that the size of aortic or pulmonary cusps in adults can vary by only a few millimeters, a graft between 17mm and 23mm in diameter is chosen according to the ring size based on the body surface area as it has already been described above [22] (Fig.9).

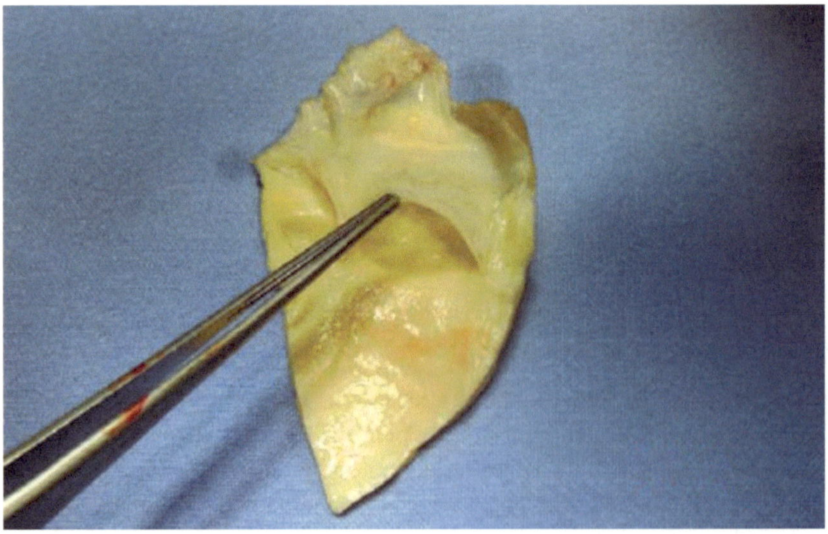

Figure 9. Aortic monocusp allograft with the anterior leaflet of the mitral valve (From Mulinari L A et al [22] with permission)

http://dx.doi.org/10.5772/57111

Technique of implantation: after inspecting the graft, one of the larger cusps is selected. Then, the graft is cut to fit a segment of the aortic or pulmonary wall that is distal to this cusp. Using a Nº 5-0 polypropylene suture, the procedure is done in such way that the cusp edge can be at the same level of the edges of the native pulmonary valve [22] (Fig 10).

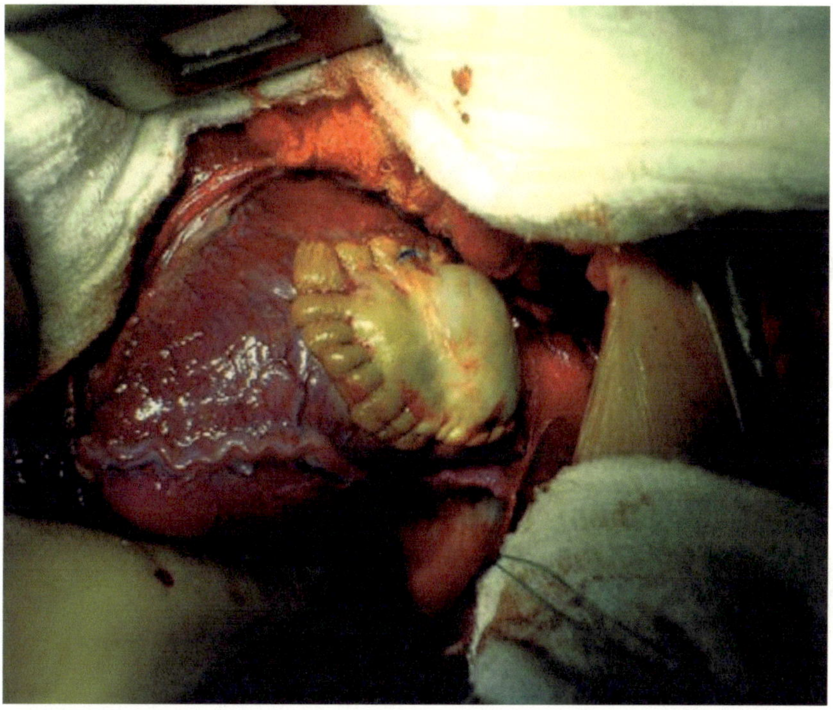

Figure 10. Pulmonary monocusp allograft implantation (From Mulinari L A et al [22] with permission)

8. Left pulmonary artery stenosis

As postulated by Kalangos et al [23] only one of the pulmonary artery branches has the same anatomical direction as the main stem of the PA, either the right or the left pulmonary artery. This particular feature is important because it can directly affect the surgical outcome; therefore, the patch enlargement technique must be performed in accordance to the anatomy of the pulmonary arch in each individual case (Fig. 11)

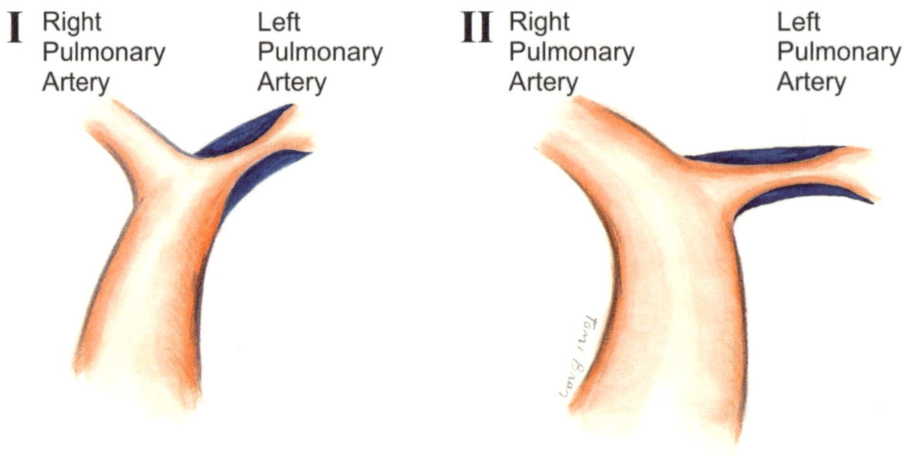

Figure 11. The pulmonary arch morphology. Please note that only one of the pulmonary artery (PA) branches has the same flow direction as the main stem of the PA, either the left PA (I) or the right PA (II) (From Kalangos A et al [23] with permission).

In most of the cases a single transannular patch enlargement extending into the LPA is sufficient to repair stenosis of the origin of the LPA when it has the same axis as the main PA (Fig. 12)

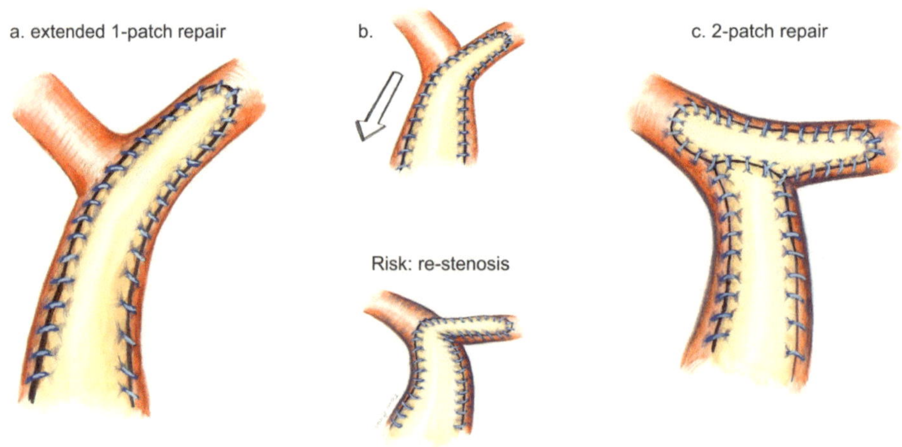

Figure 12. Reconstruction of the origin of the pulmonary artery (PA) branches for patients with left PA stenosis. (a) The left PA has the same axis as the main PA; Surgical technique: 1-patch enlargement extending into the left PA. If the right PA is the branch with the same axis as the main PA: (b) 1-patch extending into the left PA is not a suitable technique because of later risk of "kinking" which will lead to restenosis; (c) A 2-patch enlargement technique avoids the risk of "kinking" and will reduce the risk for later restenosis. (From Kalangos A et al [23] with permission).

http://dx.doi.org/10.5772/57111

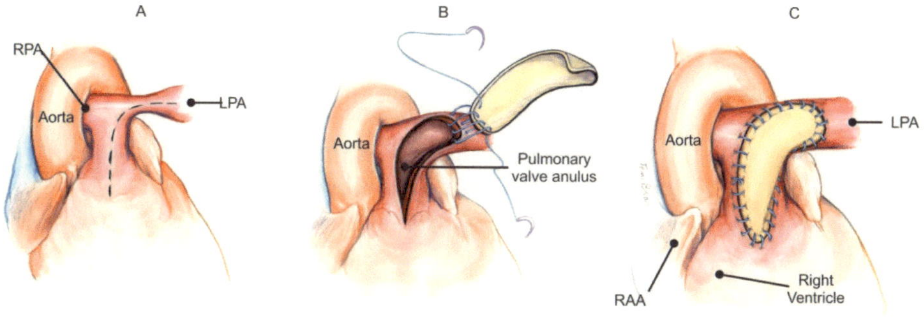

Figure 13. A- Stenosis of LPA. Dashed line indicates extent of incision. B- Single-patch repair of stenosis of LPA. C- Complete repair. Note that LPA has the same axis as the pulmonary trunk. LPA - Left pulmonary artery RPA - Right pulmonary artery

As the LPA is usually an extension of the pulmonary trunk, isololated stenosis at origin of LPA is uncommon. In these uncommon situations in which a transannular patch is not needed, an incision is made across the stenosis in the origin of the LPA and a rectangular patch of pericardium is trimmed and sewn in to place using Nº 6-0 polypropylene sutures [4,23] (Fig. 14)

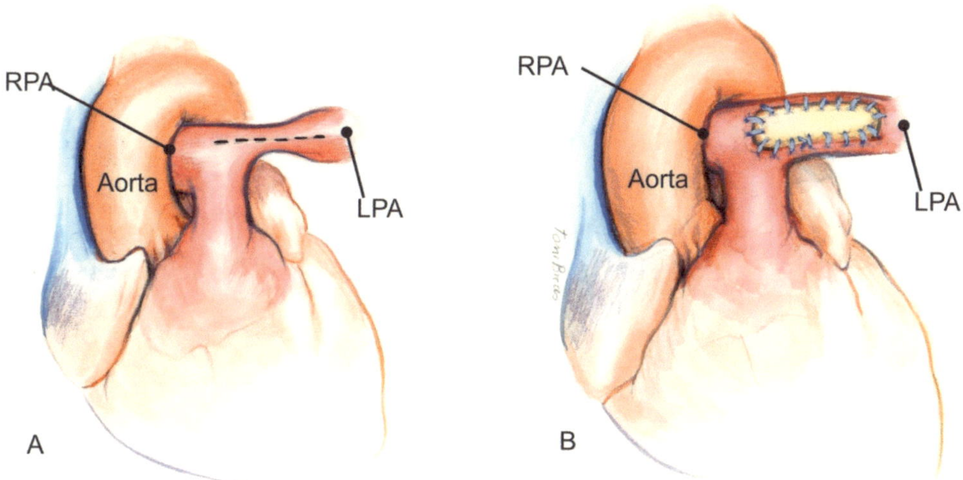

Figure 14. A- Isololated stenosis at origin of LPA. Dashed line indicates extent of incision. B- Single-patch repair at origin of LPA. LPA - Left pulmonary artery RPA - Right pulmonary artery

9. Right pulmonary artery stenosis

The RPA is usually not an extension of the pulmonary trunk but comes off its side at a right angle requiring a more complex repair than that used for stenosis of the LPA [1,15,23].

After mobilizing the aorta, the pulmonary trunk and the left and right pulmonary branches, the origin of the RPA is disconnected from the pulmonary trunk. Lateral incisions are made to enlarge the orifice in the side of the pulmonary trunk. The RPA is incised from its narrow orifice back into its wide portion. A rectangular piece of pericardium is trimmed and sewn to the RPA to make a markedly enlarged proximal RPA. The proximal end of the reconstructed RPA is then sutured to the enlarged orifice in the side of the pulmonary trunk using Nº 6-0 polypropylene sutures and closely placed sutures, while taking care to avoid any purse- string effect [4,23] (Fig.15)

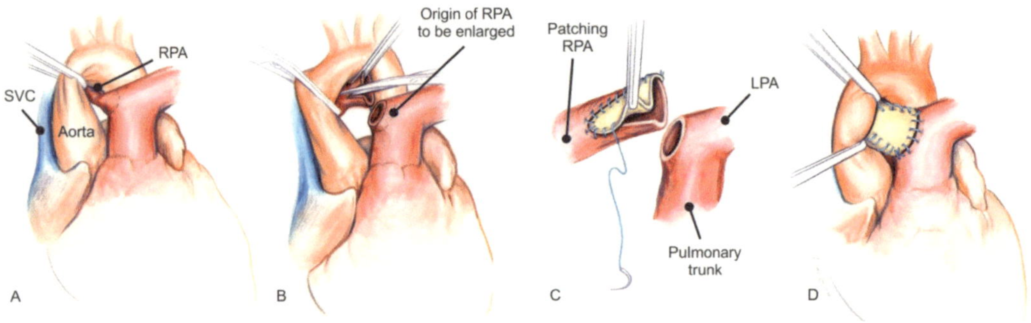

Figure 15. A- Exposure of RPA by mobilizing the aorta. B- RPA is disconnected from the pulmonary trunk. Dashed line indicates extent of incision. C- Single-patch repair of the anterior aspect of RPA. D- Re-anastomosis of the enlarged RPA to the pulmonary trunk. LPA - Left pulmonary artery RPA - Right pulmonary artery. SVC – Superior Vena Cava.

Another alternative is to suture the posterior edge of the opened RPA to the back wall of the opened pulmonary trunk. A rectangular piece of pericardium is then sewn to the remaining opening to widen it further; however, this technique is more demanding and may generate tension on the anastomosis.

Transection of the ascending aorta may improve exposure in cases of stenosis of the proximal RPA as described by Singh et al [24] (Fig.16)

http://dx.doi.org/10.5772/57111

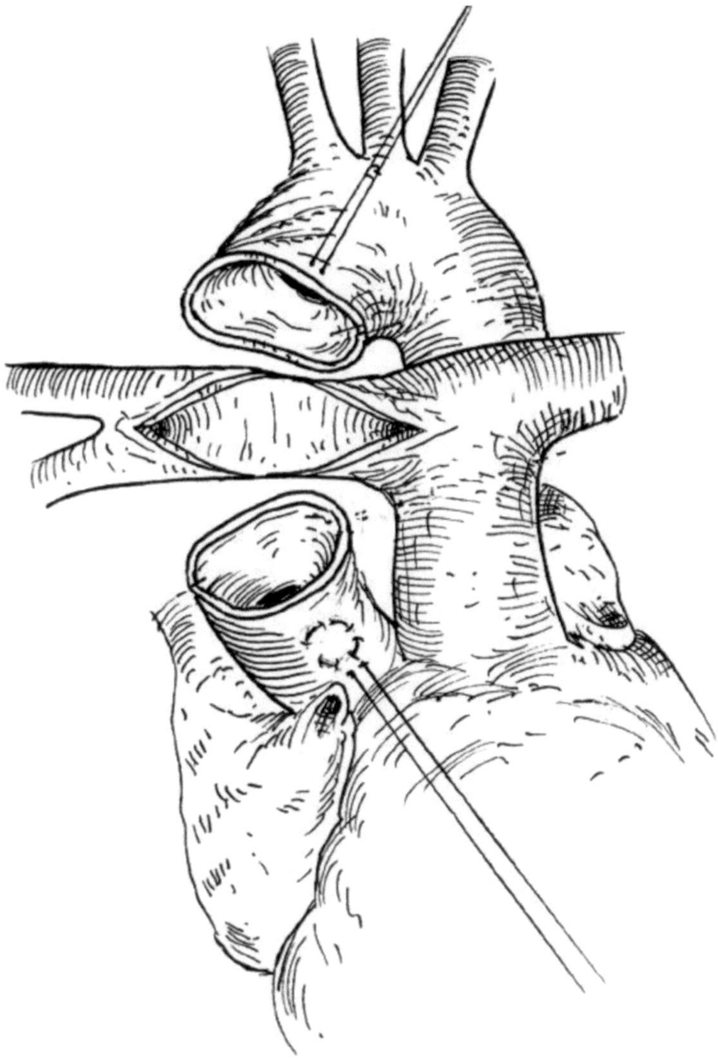

Figure 16. The ends of the transected ascending aorta retracted to expose the proximal right pulmonary artery (From Singh et al [24] with permission)

As shown in the figure above, the aortic transection facilitates exposure of the distal main PA, confluence and branches up to the hilum, especially in patients with difficult anatomy and sternal re-entry. This maneuver is recommended in patients requiring exposure of the main PA, its bifurcation, and branches during surgery for congenital heart disease, especially if adequate exposure is critical for successful repair (Fig. 17).

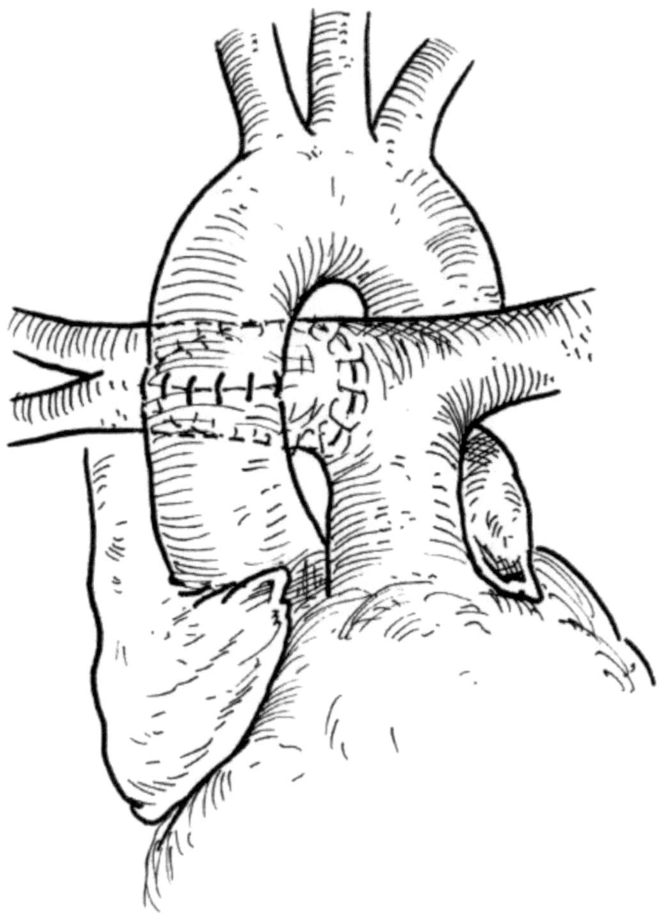

Figure 17. Completed reconstruction of the proximal right pulmonary artery and the aortic anastomosis (From Singh et al [24] with permission)

10. Bifurcation stenosis of the pulmonary trunk

The most common location of recurrent RVOT obstruction is at the pulmonary bifurcation or at the origin of the pulmonary artery branches [7,25].

Bifurcation stenosis is characterized by both LPA and RPA ostia stenosis to a similar degree and over a short distance (<15 mm) with the distal pulmonary trunk similarly narrowed making the bifurcation more Y shape than usual. However, repair of bifurcation stenosis is indicated only when the stenosis is severe [1,4,6,7,16].

The first option for infants is repair rather than replacement; however, in children age 5 years or older, the optimal procedure may be to replace the pulmonary valve, trunk, bifurcation, and proximal RPA and LPA with a pulmonary allograft [22,26,27].

Selecting the graft:

A 22- to 25-mm-diameter allograft can provide a good hemodynamic result in this complex situation. There is a trend towards the RVOT enlargement using a homologous and decellularized allograft putting forward a theoretical attempt of a graft with greater durability potential than those currently available. Decellularized grafts may be related to a lower immune response when compared with cryopreserved grafts [22, 27-32].(Fig. 18)

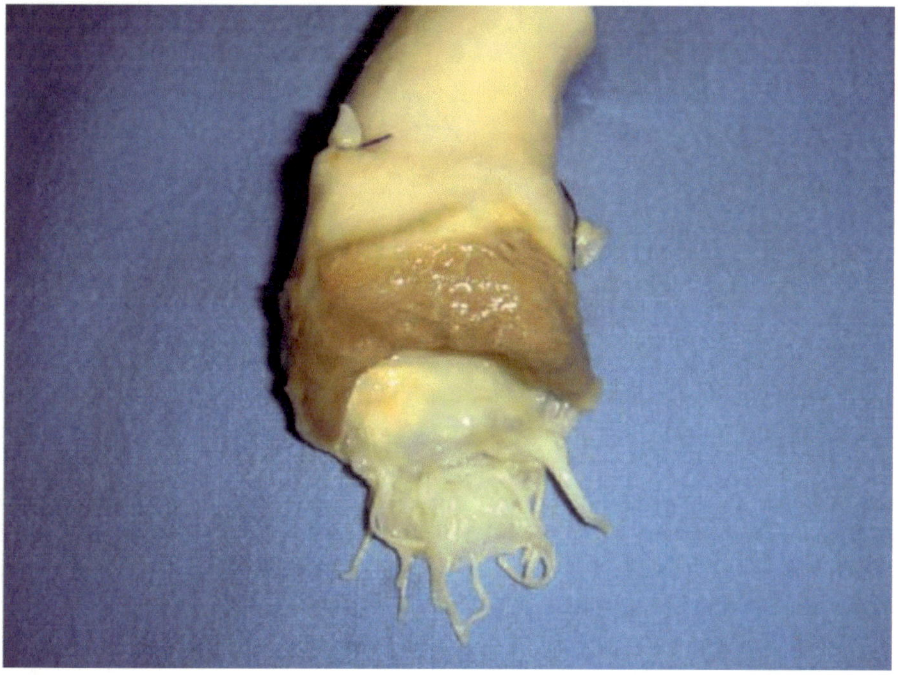

Figure 18. Decellularized aortic allograft(From Mulinari L A et al [22] with permission)

11. Surgical technique

a. Repair (for children < 5 years old)

The aortopulmonary septum is dissected and the ascending aorta is freed completely from the main PA and its branches, and then mobilized. A resection of the anterior aspect of the entire bifurcation is performed in a Y-shape fashion. The defect is repaired with a Y-shaped patch (pericardium, PTFE or allograft) using 6-0 or 7-0 absorbable sutures. (Fig. 19)

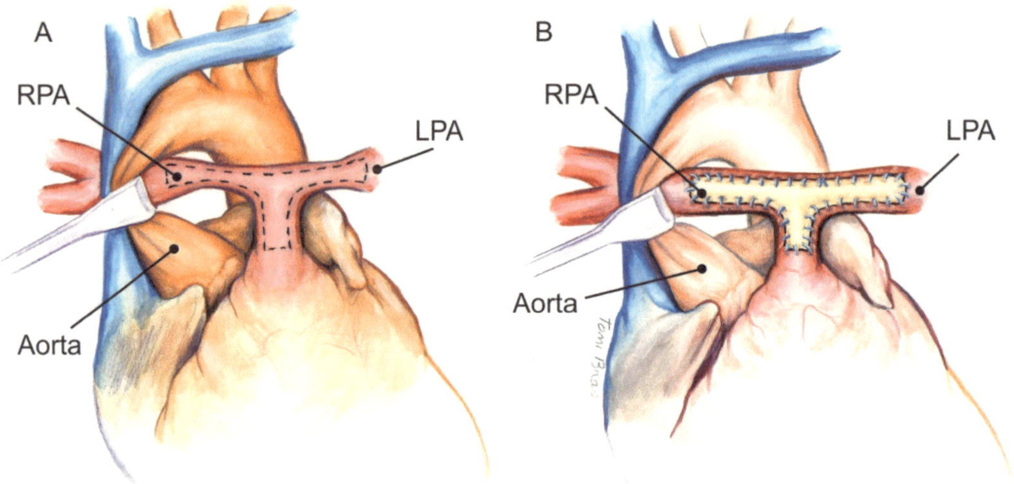

Figure 19. A- Pulmonary trunk and bifurcation stenosis. Dashed line indicates extent of incision. B- Single-Y-shape-patch repair of pulmonary artery bifurcation. LPA - Left pulmonary artery RPA - Right pulmonary artery.

b. Replacement (for children ≥ 5 years old)

The entire ascending aorta is completely freed from its posterior connections and from pulmonary trunk and its bifurcation. At this time, the ascending aorta may be divided if required [23]. The superior vena cava is completely mobilized and the RPA and LPA are dissected to the point where the first branch is visualized and subsequently transected beyond the narrow areas. A vertical ventriculotomy is carried across the annulus into the pulmonary trunk which is ultimately transected.

A 22- to 25-mm-diameter allograft can provide a good hemodynamic result in this complex situation.

Distal anastomoses are made first with continuous Nº 5-0 or 6-0 polypropylene suture. The proximal conduit anastomosis is made by commencing the suturing posteriorly where the allograft is opposed to the superior margin of the ventriculotomy using an Nº 4-0 polypropylene suture. The suture line is continued from the midline along both sides around about half the circumference of the conduit, and the sutures are held. A patch of pericardium 2 to 5 mm larger than the diameter of the allograft valve annulus is cut to an approximate semilunar shape and sutured into place to complete the anterior half of the anastomosis serving as a roof on the ventriculotomy incision and preventing the graft distortion. [4,22,32] (Fig. 20)

http://dx.doi.org/10.5772/57111

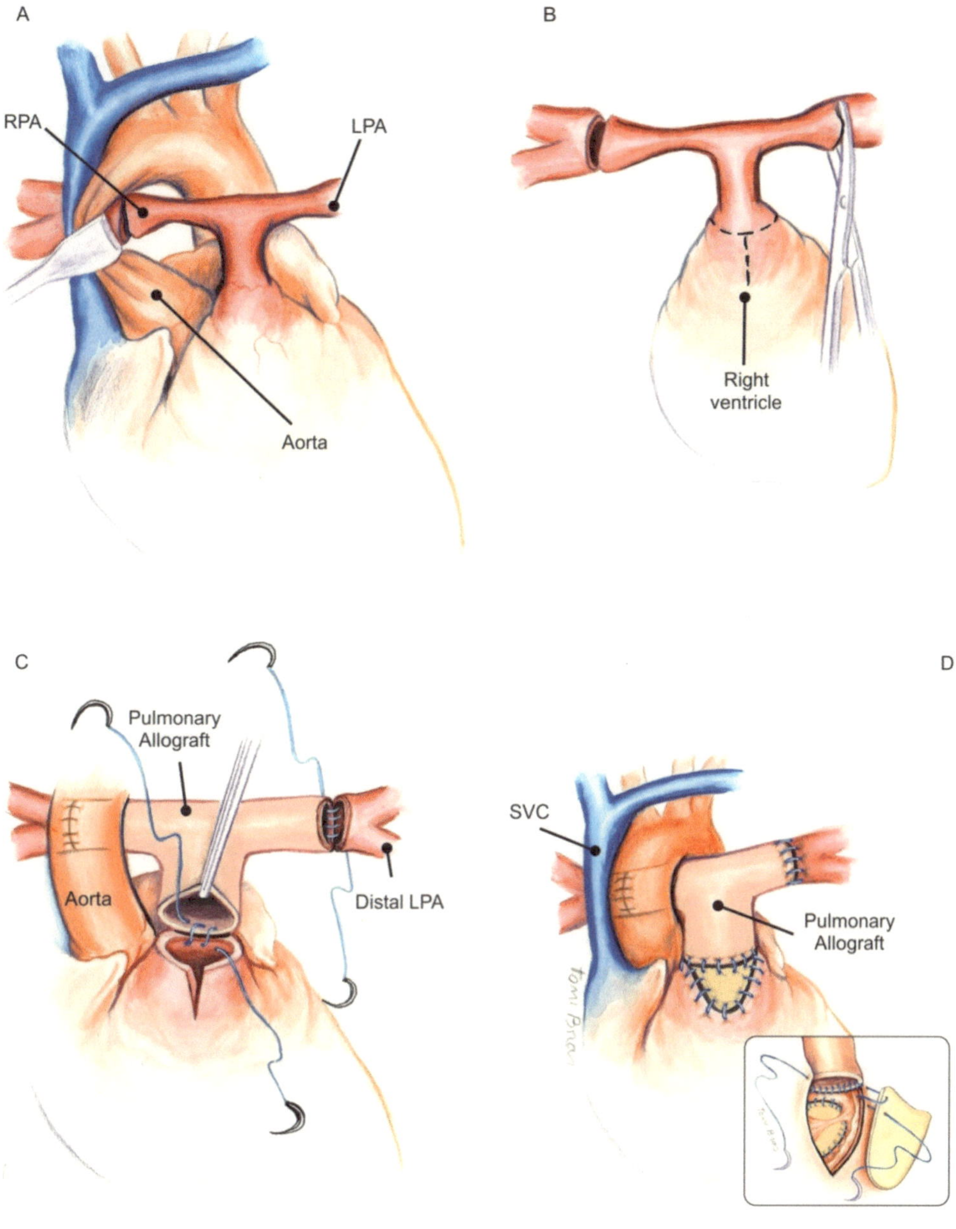

Figure 20. A- Pulmonary trunk and bifurcation stenosis. B- Resection of pulmonary trunk and its bifurcation. Dashed line indicates extent of resection. C- Replacement of pulmonary bifurcation with interposition of a pulmonary allograft. D- Completion of the replacement. Note the insertion of a pericardial roof on the ventriculotomy to prevent allograft distortion (inlet). LPA - Left pulmonary artery RPA - Right pulmonary artery. SVC – Superior Vena Cava.

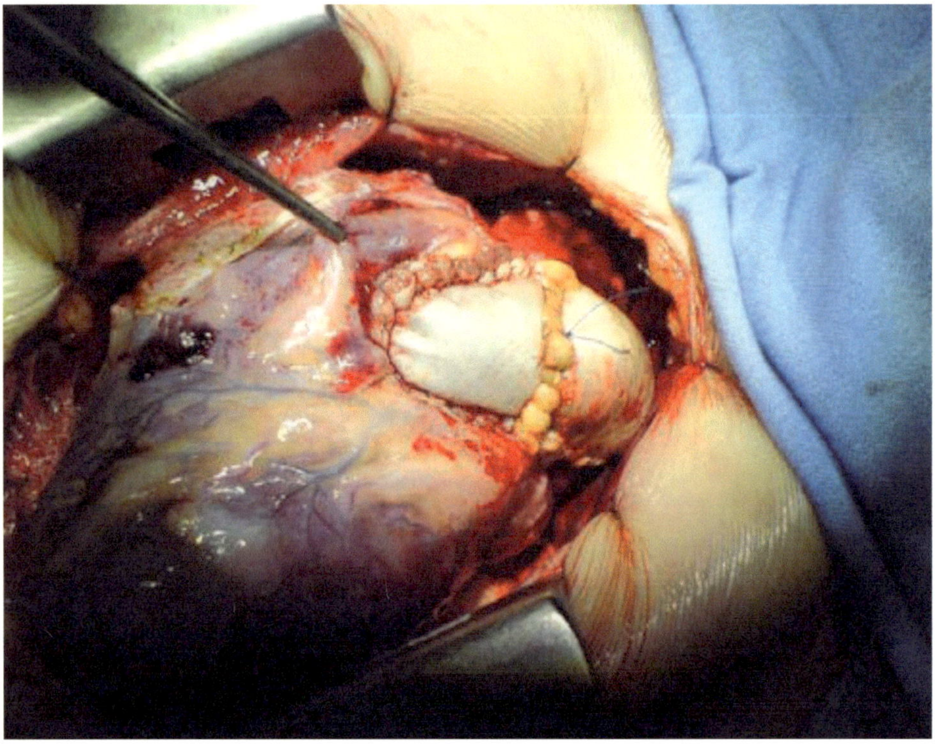

Figure 21. Pulmonary allograft implantation with bovine pericardium extension (From Mulinari L A et al [22] with permission)

12. Special remarks

- Isolated LPA and RPA stenosis in TOF requires distinct surgical repair otherwise a residual stenosis or arterial kinking may occur.
- Replacement of the entire pulmonary bifurcation must be reserved for children 5 years of age and over with severe bifurcation stenosis for whom allograft insertion seems to be the best option.
- Decellularized allograft for patching and also as a conduit is a promising alternative for reconstruction of the pulmonary trunk and its branches in TOF
- If a conduit insertion is required, care must be taken to position it nearly in the same position as a normal pulmonary artery by directing it toward the patient`s left shoulder as it come off the right ventriculotomy in order to prevent compression by the sternum.
- Although the growth potential of pedicled pericardium has not been clearly demonstrated, it is a very attractive alternative for enlargement of small pulmonary arteries or the RVOT in TOF or pulmonary atresia because it maintains its native vascular and neural supply

which may avoid further reoperations to replace the pulmonary arterial trunk with an extracardiac conduit after growth of the child.

- Postoperative RV/LV ratio ≥ 0.9 indicates residual obstruction either muscular or arterial, which must be promptly surgically removed or ameliorated by percutaneous balloon dilatation, if possible.

Author details

Vinicius José da Silva Nina

Cardiac Surgery Unit, University Hospital of the Federal University of Maranhão, Brazil

References

[1] Anderson RH, Weinberg PM: *The clinical anatomy of tetralogy of Fallot*. Cardiology in the Young 2005, 15 (Suppl 1):38-47.

[2] Bailliard F, Anderson R H. *Tetralogy of Fallot: Review*. Orphanet Journal of Rare Diseases 2009, 4:2

[3] Apitz C, Webb G D, Redington A N. *Tetralogy of Fallot: Seminar*. Lancet 2009; 374: 1462–71.

[4] Kouchoukos NT, Blackstone EH, Doty DB, Hanley FL, Karp RB. *Ventricular septal defect with pulmonary stenosis or atresia.* In: Kirklin/Barratt-Boyes cardiac surgery: morphology, diagnostic criteria, natural history, techniques, results, and indications. Churchill Livingstone, 3rd edition, 2003, pp: 946-1073.

[5] Elzenga NJ, von Suylen RJ, Froh-Mulder I, Essed CE, Bos E, Quaegebeur JM. *Juxtaductal pulmonary artery coarctation. An underestimated cause of branch pulmonary artery stenosis in patients with pulmonary atresia or stenosis and a ventricular septal defect.* J Thorac Cardiovasc Surg 1990; 100: 416-24.

[6] Shimazaki Y, Blackstone EH, Kirklin JW, Jonas RA, Mandell V, Colvin EV. *The dimensions of the right venricular outflow tract and and pulmonary arteries in tetralogy of Fallot and pulmonary stenosis.* J Thorac Cardiovasc Surg 1992; 103: 692-705.

[7] Fraser Jr C D, Latson L A, Mee R B B. *Surgical repair of severe bilateral branch pulmonary artery stenosis*. Ann Thorac Surg 1995;59:738-40.

[8] Fellows KE, Smith J, Keane JF. *Preoperative angiocardiography in infants with tetrad of Fallot. Review of 36 cases*. Am J Cardiol 1981; 47: 1279-85.

[9] Hoohenkerk GJ, Schoof PH, Bruggemans EF, Rijlaarsdam M, Hazekamp MG: *28 years' experience with transatrial-transpulmonary repair of atrioventricular septal defect with tetralogy of Fallot*. Ann Thorac Surg 2008, 85(5):1686-1689.

[10] Stewart RD, Backer CL, Young L, Mavroudis C: *Tetralogy of Fallot: Results of a pulmonary valve-sparing strategy*. Ann Thorac Surg 2005; 80:1431-1439.

[11] Agnoletti G, Boudjemline Y, Bonnet D, Sidi D, Vouhé P. *Surgical reconstruction of occluded pulmonary arteries in patients with congenital heart disease: effects on pulmonary artery growth*. Circulation 2004;109:2314 - 2318.

[12] Shinkawa T, Yamagishi M, Shuntoh K, Miyazaki T, Hisaoka T, Yaku H. *Pulmonary arterial reconstruction for pulmonary coarctation in early infancy*. Ann Thorac Surg 2007; 83:188–92.

[13] Kaneko Y, Okabe H, Nagata N, Ohuchi H, Kobayashi J, Kanemoto S, ItohK. *Lay-open pulmonary arterioplasty for postoperative hilar pulmonary artery stenosis*. J Thorac Cardiovasc Surg 1997;114:406-12.

[14] Rowlatt UF, Rimoldi HJA, Lev M *The quantitative anatomy of the normal child`s heart*. Pediatr Clin North Am 1963; 10: 499-588.

[15] De la Cruz MV, Anselmi G, Romero A, Monroy GA *A qualitative and quantitative study of the ventricles and great vessels of normal children*. Am Heart J 1960; 60: 675-690.

[16] Capps SB, Elkins RC, Fronk DM.*Body surface area as a predictor of aortic and pulmonary valve diameter.* J Thorac Cardiovasc Surg. 2000;119(5):975-82.

[17] Jacob M F F B, De Marchi C H, Croti U A, Braile DM *Atrioventricular septal defect with tetralogy of Fallot in patient with Down's syndrome. Rev Bras Cir Cardiovasc 2009; 24(3): 422-424*

[18] Croti UA, Braile D M, Moscardini A C, Kozak M F.*Enlargement of the right ventricular outflow tract using autologous pediculated pericardium in the tetralogy of fallot treatment. Rev Bras Cir Cardiovasc 2008; 23(4): 583-585*

[19] Khoury W, Lang-Lazdunski L, Vernant F, Thibert M, Leca F. *Pedicled pericardium for repair of right ventricular outflow tract and pulmonary arterial stenoses in tetralogy of Fallot: a six-year experience.* J Thorac Cardiovasc Surg 1996;112:424-32.

[20] Lukács L, Záborszky B, Sárközy K, Aŕvay A. *Reconstruction of the right ventricular outflow tract with bovine pericardial monocusp patch.* Tex Heart Inst J 1984; 11(3): 234–237.

[21] Maluf M A. *Late outcome of right ventricular outflow tract repair using bicuspid pulmonary prosthesis in tetralogy of Fallot surgery repair: case report. Rev Bras Cir Cardiovasc 2009; 24(4): 574-577*

[22] Mulinari L A, Navarro F B, PimenteL G K, Miyazaki S M, Binotto C N, Pelissari E C, Miyague N I, Da Costa F D A. *The use and midium-term evaluation of decellularized allog-*

raft cusp in the surgical treatment of the Tetralogy of Fallot. Rev Bras Cir Cardiovasc 2008; 23(2): 197-203

[23] Faidutti B, Christenson J T, Beghetti M, Friedli B, Kalangos A. *How to diminish reoperation rates after initial repair of tetralogy of Fallot?* Ann Thorac Surg 2002;73:96 –101

[24] Singh A, Krishnan G S, Agarwal R, Dave D, Kotturathu M. *Ascending Aortic Transection: Useful Adjunct in Pulmonary Artery Reconstruction. Asian Cardiovasc Thorac Ann 2008;16:254–5*

[25] Oechslin EN, Harrisson DA, Harris L, *et al. Reoperation in adults with repair of tetralogy of Fallot: indications and outcomes.* J Thorac Cardiovasc Surg 1999;118:245–51.

[26] Burczynski PL, McKay R, Arnold R, Mitchell DR, Sabino GP. *Homograft replacement of the pulmonary artery bifurcation. J Thorac Cardiovasc Surg 1989; 98:623-31.*

[27] Clarke DR, Campbell DN, Pappas G. *Pulmonary allograft conduit repair of tetralogy of Fallot. An alternative to transannular patch repair. J Thorac Cardiovasc Surg 1989; 98:730-6; discussion 736-7.*

[28] Hopkins RA, Jones AL, Wolfinbarger L, Moore MA, Bert AA, Lofland GK. *Decellularization reduces calcification while improving both durability and 1-year functional results of pulmonary homograft valves in juvenile sheep. J Thorac Cardiovasc Surg.* 2009;137(4): 907-13.

[29] Bechtel JF, Müller-Steinhardt M, Schmidtke C, Brunswik A, Stierle U, Sievers HH. *Evaluation of the decellularized pulmonary valve homograft (SynerGraft).* J Heart Valve Dis.2003;12(6):734-9.

[30] Hawkins JA, Hillman ND, Lambert LM, Jones J, Di Russo GB, Profaizer T, *et al. Immunogenicity of decellularized cryopreserved allografts in pediatric cardiac surgery:comparison with standard cryopreserved allografts*. J Thorac Cardiovasc Surg. 2003;126(1):247-52.

[31] da Costa FD, Dohmen PM, Duarte D, von Glenn C, Lopes SV, Haggi Filho H, *et al. Immunological and echocardiographic evaluation of decellularized versus cryopreserved allografts during the Ross operation.* Eur J Cardiothorac Surg. 2005;27(4):572-8.

[32] Costa F, Fornazari DF, Matsuda CN, Torres RA, Sardetto E,Ferreira ADA, *et al. Ten years experience of aortic valve replacement with aortic homograft root replacement.* Rev Bras Cir Cardiovasc. 2006;21(2):155-64.

Chapter 10

Adjustable Pulmonary Artery Banding

Renato S. Assad

Additional information is available at the end of the chapter

http://dx.doi.org/10.5772/57117

1. Introduction

Pulmonary trunk banding is a technique of palliative surgical therapy. It has been used as a staged approach to operative correction for children born with cardiac defects characterized by left-to-right shunting or in need for ventricle retraining. This technique can be used to somehow diminish pulmonary overcirculation or to promote myocardial hypertrophy until subsequent total repair be possible. It consists of placing a band well proximal to the pulmonary artery (PA) bifurcation. The band is tightened and secured by suture to narrow the main PA, until the pressure distal to the band is one-third to one-half that of the aorta. Excessive blood flow to the lungs is therefore diminished by constricting the PA circumference, thereby achieving the desired limitation of the pulmonary flow and a balance with aortic blood flow. Nevertheless, skill and accuracy of the surgery, supplemented by good fortune are most likely to assure success in this imprecise conventional procedure. In addition, the band commonly used is fixed and unchanged in the postoperative course. It means that adjustment of the traditional band is unpredictable and empiric, performed under artificial conditions, different from the postoperative period. Since mid-80's, early definitive intracardiac repair has largely replaced palliation with PA banding. This trend has evolved because many centers have demonstrated improved outcomes with primary corrective surgery as an initial intervention in the neonate with congenital heart disease. Although the use of PA banding has recently decreased significantly, it continues to maintain a therapeutic role in certain subsets of patients with congenital heart disease. PA banding may be applicable to the very sick and small infants with torrential pulmonary blood flow, commonly producing heart failure beyond age one to two months, when diminished pulmonary vascular resistance allows substantial left-to-right shunting. Babies usually have feeding difficulties and failure to gain weight and grow. Multiple muscular ventricular septal defects with a "Swiss cheese" septum, single or multiple ventricular septal defects with coarctation of the aorta or interrupted aortic arch, single ventricle type of defects with increased pulmonary blood flow, are among the lesions in which the use of PA banding may allow time for recovery until the patient can be submitted to definitive surgery.

PA banding has also played a role in the preparation and "training" of the left ventricle (LV) in patients with d-transposition of the great arteries (TGA) that are evaluated for a delayed arterial switch procedure (Jatene procedure). It has also been applied in patients with congenitally corrected TGA (CCTGA) or after Senning or Mustard operations with right ventricular (RV) failure. It is now recognized that the arterial switch operation can be done only with a LV conditioned to pump against systemic resistance. After birth, the LV starts pumping blood against the progressive low-resistance pulmonary vasculature, while the RV assumes the systemic function, and also the necessary muscle mass, to overcome a higher vascular resistance. These significant differences in LV and RV muscle mass progress over time and may assume considerable importance if the LV is suddenly required to perform against systemic vascular resistance, as in the arterial switch operation. For the majority of the patients with TGA referred beyond the neonatal period, who presents with an intact (or virtually intact) ventricular septum, the LV cannot retain pressure close to systemic levels. It is important to take advantage of these anatomic features during the neonatal period, in which LV is still adequate to handle systemic circulation, to carry out the arterial switch operation in a "safe" period. A number of circumstances can arise, causing postponement of surgery beyond the neonatal period. For example, a neonate may be seriously ill with necrotizing enterocolitis, renal or hepatic failure, or a hemorrhage in the central nervous system. Also, the neonate may be geographically distant from a center offering the arterial switch operation.

The establishment of the arterial switch operation as the best option for the surgical treatment of TGA, as well as the well-studied concept about the RV's inability to maintain appropriate performance as a long-term systemic ventricle in atrial inversion operations or in CTTGA, led many centers to retrain the hypotrophied LV, aiming to surgically recruit it for systemic circulation. Therefore, arterial switch operation must be performed after preliminary PA banding, with or without a systemic to PA shunt, to stimulate the development of LV muscle mass, followed by an arterial switch operation later on, a concept introduced by Yacoub et al. in 1977. The retraining period between the two stages will allow the LV to function as a systemic pump. Some years later, the Boston Children's Hospital group introduced the concept of rapid, two-stage arterial switch operation for TGA, limiting the interval between the first and the second operation to an average of seven days. However, one of the greatest limitations of this technical approach was related to the lack of adjustability of the PA banding. The degree of PA banding may be inadequate or imprecise and can cause an important acute systolic overload of the LV. That trial succeeded in their objective, once there was significant cardiac mass acquisition in about 7 days, reducing the risks of complications resulted from the primary repair of TGA in a patient with unprepared LV. However, the "rapid approach" produced some degree of unsatisfactory myocardial contractile performance in the late follow-up of about one fourth of the patients. In addition, other centers have reported a high morbidity and mortality rates associated to that 2-stage approach. Experimental studies have demonstrated myocardial edema and necrosis in hearts that experience abrupt systolic overload, followed by late ventricular failure. That is why the use of an adjustable PA banding system for LV retraining to this subset of patients became of interest to many investigators. Since then, several studies have been carried out to achieve the most physiologic way to obtain LV retraining.

In developing countries, the number of patients with TGA presenting beyond the neonatal period is still considerable. The rapid 2-stage approach remains an interesting alternative for that population with late referral. Nevertheless, preliminary traditional banding of the pulmonary trunk may cause the following problems: (1) Imprecision of optimal occlusion may occur at the time of banding; (2) additional palliative procedures may be necessary to increase pulmonary blood flow; (3) anatomic distortion of the pulmonary trunk, pulmonary arteries, or both may occur. (4) The degree of abrupt acute systolic overload on the left ventricle may impair late ventricular function.

Said that, it sounds like traditional PA banding, used to treat the above-mentioned heart lesions, is inconvenient in that it does not allow late and fine adjustment according to the patient's clinical condition over time, and therefore sometimes requiring new interventions to achieve that.

2. Historical notes of adjustable PA banding systems

The idea of adjustable banding device composed of a hydraulic cuff and a self-sealing button was first proposed in 1957. In fact, Jacobson & McAllister proposed a device consisted of a rubber cuff, with a lateral opening, and connected to a reservoir protected by self-sealing rubber (Figure 1). It was used on the great vessels of dogs, aiming a congestive heart failure model. Complications in handling the device were observed.

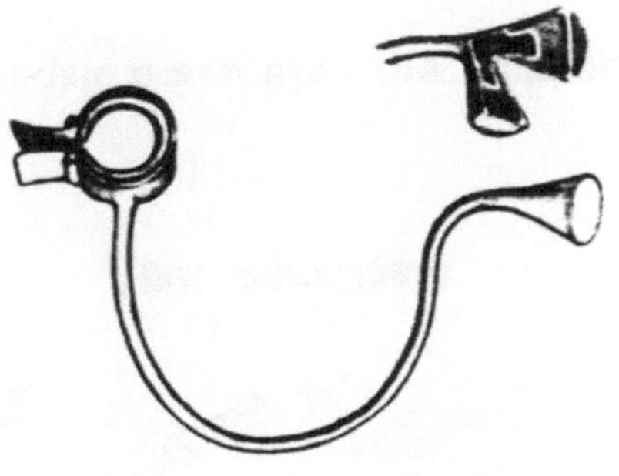

Figure 1. Jacobson & McAllister proposed in 1957 a device consisted of a rubber cuff, with a lateral opening, and connected to a reservoir protected by self-sealing rubber

In 1969, Bishop & Cole improved Jacobson & McAllister device by covering the cuff with silicone, with the aim of reducing local tissue reaction (Figure 2). They induced RV hypertrophy and congestive heart failure in a dog model.

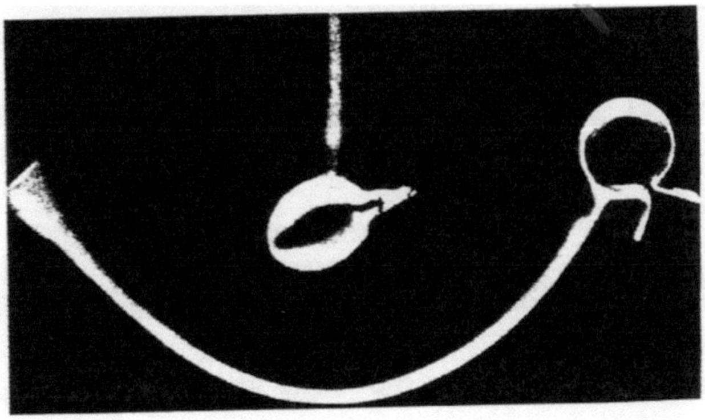

Figure 2. In 1969, Bishop & Cole device was covered with silicone to reduce tissue reaction

In 1972, Edmunds et al introduced two main changes: an external, non-deformable layer on the hydraulic cuff and silicone, instead of rubber (Figure 3). However, they observed asymmetric inflation or rupture of the cuff, and leakage of the injected material prevented from clinical use.

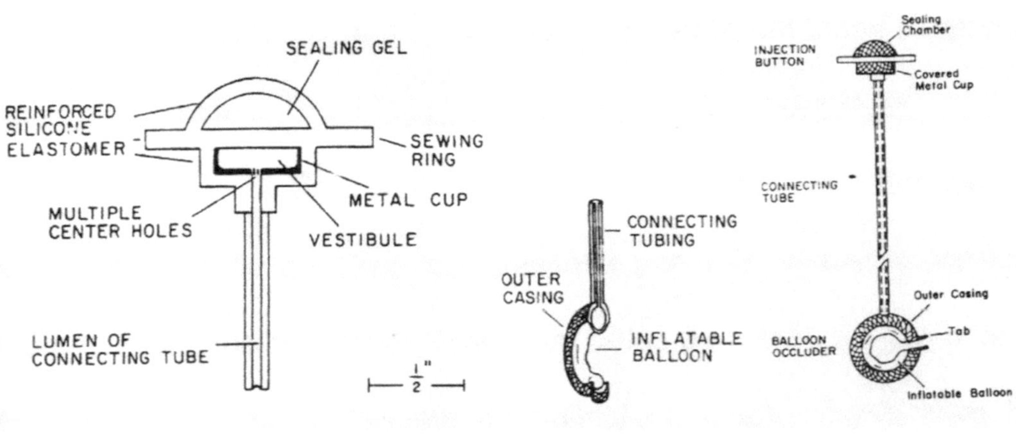

Figure 3. In 1972, Edmunds prototype presented an external, non-deformable layer on the hydraulic cuff and silicone, instead of rubber

In 1985, a new device made of biologically stable material (medical grade silicone) was introduced by Park et al. (Figure 4) The cuff was covered with reinforced braid and coated with silicone. The self-sealing button has a silicone diaphragm which did enable repeated needle puncture, avoiding leaking through the button. The device implanted in dogs and lambs was easily and effectively adjusted.

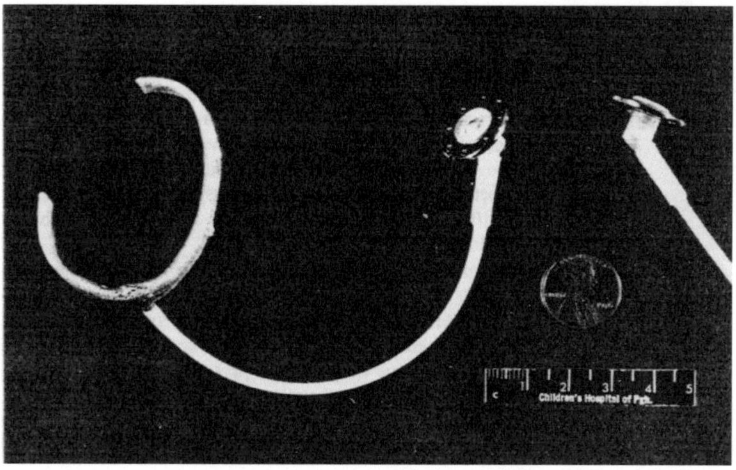

Figure 4. In 1985, Park introduced a prototype made of medical grade silicone. The cuff was covered with reinforced braid and coated with silicone. The self-sealing button had a silicone diaphragm which did enable repeated needle puncture.

During that same year, Solis et al. proposed a similar device to the previous one, intended to prepare the subpulmonary ventricle for the two-stage Jatene operation for the first time in the literature (Figure 5). Nevertheless, when the system was submitted to a high pressure gradient, as in the systemic circulation, dilation of the reservoir and the connecting tube occurred. In addition, there was a tendency of the cuff to bulge laterally under high pressure.

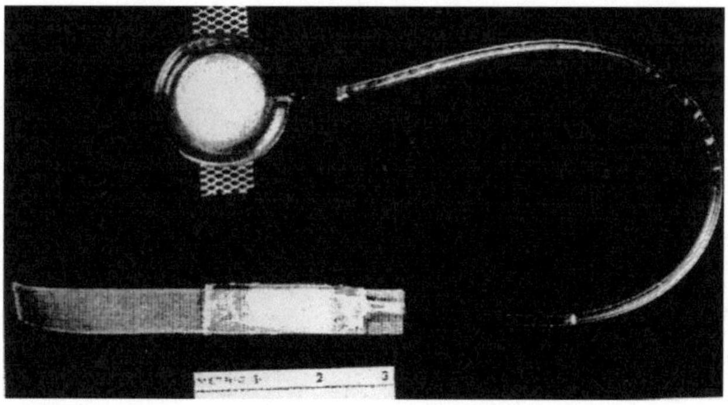

Figure 5. For the first time in the literature, Solis proposed in 1985 a similar device to prepare the subpulmonary ventricle for the two-stage Jatene operation.

In another study, the same group improved the strength of the material by reinforcing the cuff and the connecting tube with a spiral of 4-0 silk to withstand systemic arterial pressure. Again, they experienced bulging of the cuff due to a losing silk.

3. Adjustable PA banding system for ventricle retraining

We have begun this research line for more than two decades ago, using a balloon catheter to induce rapid pulmonary ventricular hypertrophy. We developed an experimental model of young goats, designed to adjust PA banding percutaneously. The main idea is that systolic overload might be less acute and intense using such a device than a traditional PAB, in which no changes are possible during ventricular retraining. We have assessed, by means of echocardiography and cell morphology, the behavior of the right ventricle (RV) submitted to progressive pressure load imposed by a balloon catheter positioned above the pulmonary valve. The catheter is a modification of the Swan-Ganz catheter, in which the temperature probe was removed and the respective port was annulled. The length of the catheter was shortened so that the distal orifice was placed 30 mm away from the original proximal orifice. The original balloon was replaced by a manufactured balloon made with segmented polyether polyurethane copolymer, diluted in N,N-dimethylacetamide (Figure 6).

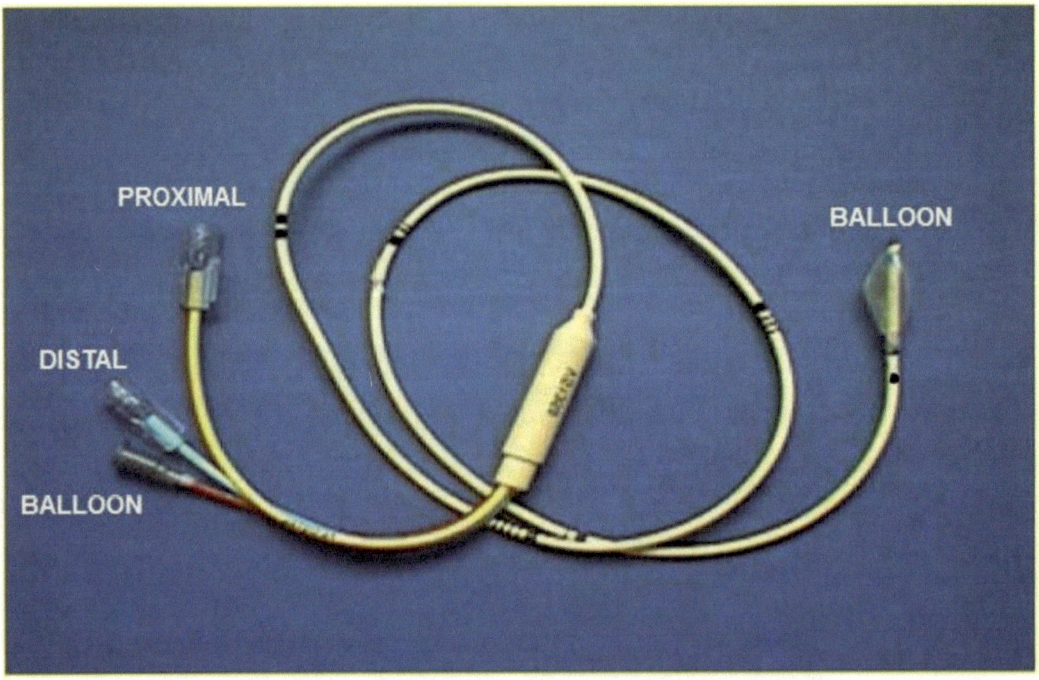

Figure 6. Balloon catheter prototype, modified from the Swan-Ganz catheter and used for subpulmonary ventricle retraining.

A rapid RV hypertrophy was achieved in a short period of six to 10 days. It has been demonstrated that nonsurgical preparation of the "pulmonary ventricle" for the 2-stage arterial switch operation could be probably accomplished non-invasively with a balloon catheter within a very few days.

http://dx.doi.org/10.5772/57117

In mid-90's, we started to study experimentally an extravascular adjustable PA banding device, with a hydraulic cuff system, connected to a self-sealing button for percutaneous systolic overload adjustment (Figure 7). The banding ring (Hazen Everett Co) is a C-shaped hydraulic cuff with a 10-mm internal diameter and a 5-mm width. Its outer layer consists of 1-mm-thick rigid silicone, which keeps it from deforming. The inner surface has a deformable layer of silicone, which expands, compressing the lumen of the vessel according to the volume injected into the inflation button. At the 2 ends of the cuff, there are small orifices that are used for securing the ring to the PA. The extension tube, also made of silicone, links the banding ring with the insufflation button. It has a 2-mm inner diameter and is 25 cm long. The inflation button (Bard Access System) is a circular reservoir made of self-sealing silicone, the base of which includes a metal plate. The reservoir has a port, which is connected to the extension tube. This button is implanted subcutaneously, thus permitting percutaneous inflation or deflation of the banding ring.

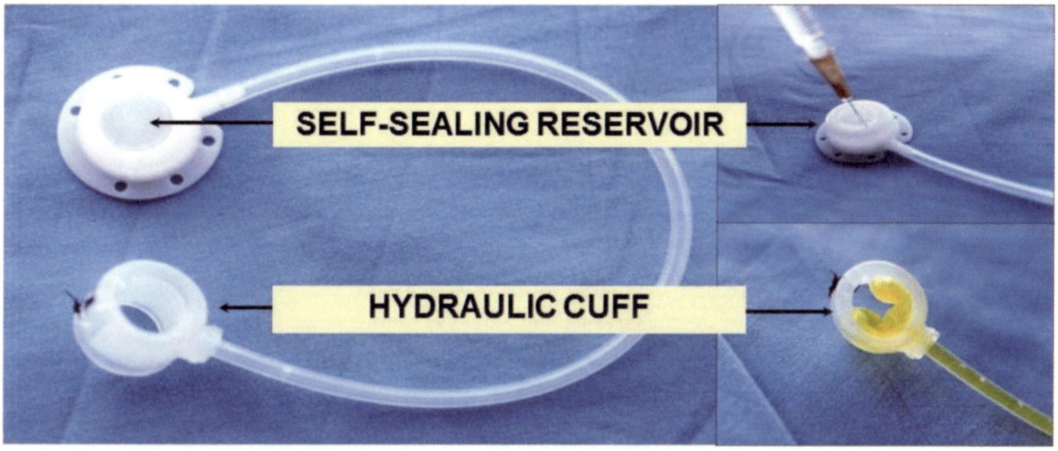

Figure 7. Adjustable banding device consisting of 3 parts: banding ring (hydraulic cuff), extension tube, and self-sealing inflation button (reservoir).

The device was implanted on the pulmonary trunk of young goats and inflated so that a 0.7 RV to LV pressure ratio was achieved. Continuous systolic overload was maintained during a 96-hour period. The study group showed a 74% increase in RV mass when compared with the control group, while a 66% increase in RV wall thickness was found by serial 2-D echocardiography. There was a 24% increase in the mean myocyte perimeter, and the myocyte area increased 61% (Figure 8).

This extravascular device was further compared to the endovascular approach (balloon catheter), during a 96-hour protocol of continuous systolic overload. Both approaches were able to induce rapid RV hypertrophy of similar magnitude (Figure 9).

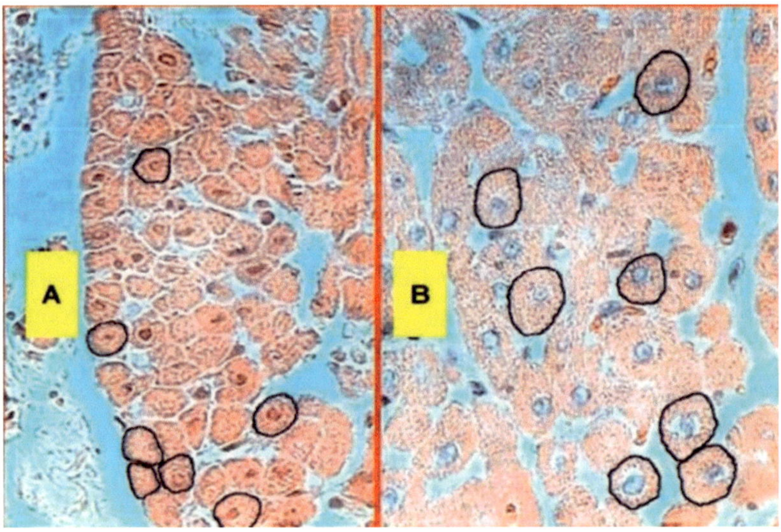

Figure 8. Microphotography of RV cardiac myocytes of animal 6 sectioned transversely at the level of the nucleus, indicating their perimeters and respective areas: A, baseline samplings; B, samplings after 96 hours of systolic overload. (Original magnification 400x)

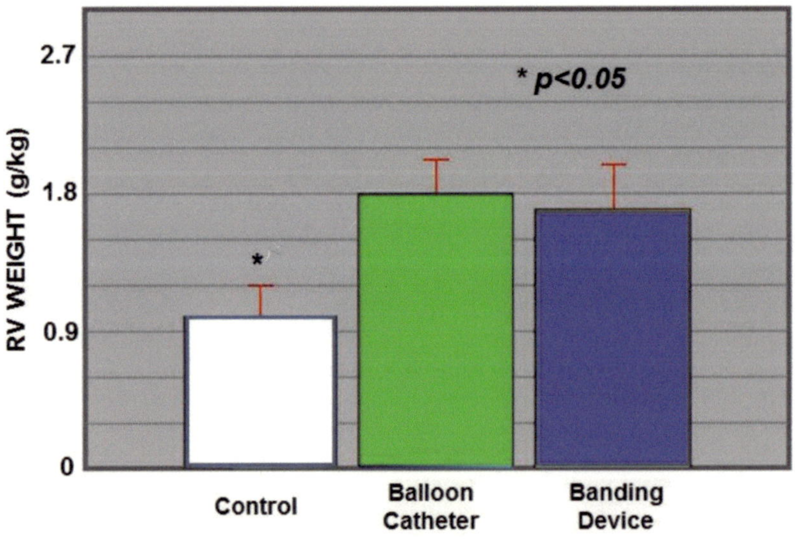

Figure 9. Both devices are able to induce a similar degree of RV hypertrophy during a 96-hour study period.

4. Intermittent systolic overload

Heart hypertrophy is the main adaptive response of a heart submitted to physiological or pathological overload. At present, there is great concern about the quality of ventricular hypertrophy, leading to questions regarding the most efficient and physiologic training program and the adaptive mechanisms involved in the process. On the other hand, the hypertrophy of an athlete's heart, characterized by normal or increased capillary density with little or no fibrosis, is a consequence of physiologic stresses like endurance exercise, intermittent by nature. It is interesting to note that the acquisition of LV mass during physical conditioning of athletes who practice swimming for example, reaches a peak in about only one week of training. Then the LV mass remains relatively constant. Based on the fact that both the cardiac and the skeletal muscles are striated, it has been proposed that a fitness program similar to that developed by athletes would lead to an acquired muscular mass with better performance. Besides that, the knowledge that the myocardium is a postmitotic organ, which means that cardiomyocytes are capable of proliferating after the neonatal period, leads to the hypothesis that myocyte hyperplasia may be an important feature in mass acquisition, although it has not been clarified to what extent it occurs. Trying to improve the rapid hypertrophic process without causing injury to the myocardium of the subpulmonary ventricle, we tried to find an analogy between the physiological hypertrophic processes with intermittent PA banding, where periods of systolic overload were alternated with resting periods of the subpulmonary ventricle. We formed a hypothesis that submitting the RV to daytime systolic overload, paired with nighttime resting period, could cause a more beneficial hypertrophic process, similar to a fitness program of athletes. We then carried out an experimental study designed to evaluate two protocols of PA banding (continuous and intermittent) and to analyze histologically the structural phenotype changes (hypertrophy and/or hyperplasia) of the contractile (cardiomyocytes) and noncontractile cells (vascular and interstitial) from the stimulated ventricle of young goats (Figure 10).

An interesting finding in this study was that both groups presented with significant increase in the RV free wall thickness. Nevertheless, this increase was significantly greater in the Intermittent Group (132.1%), compared to a 63.7% increase of in the Continuous Group. Regarding RV mass, there was a significant increase in the both groups, as compared to the Control Group (55.6% for the Continuous Group and 88.9% for the Intermittent Group), while only the Intermittent Group developed a significant increase of septal mass (40%), when compared to the Control Group (Figure 11). That study has demonstrated that intermittent systolic overload was more efficient in promoting the increase in RV mass than in the Continuous Group, considering the greater septal hypertrophy.

Morphometric analysis revealed that for both stimulated groups, hypertrophy and hyperplasia of cardiomyocytes occurred (Figure 12). Nevertheless, it is well recognized that interstitial cell proliferation is also a feature in myocardial hypertrophy caused by other factors. The interstitium has important functions, such as support for cardiomyocytes, blood and lymphatic vessels; acting as a defense mechanism against microorganisms; facilitating myocardial nutrient exchanges; and aiding in cell contraction. However, when interstitium enlargement is excessive, it may cause early diastolic dysfunction and, in the final stages, also jeopardizes systolic function. In that study, no significant difference existed in RV collagen area fraction among the three groups (Continuous, Intermittent, and Control groups). We cannot rule out the possibility that the observation time (96-hour protocol) was not sufficient to demonstrate an increase in the interstitial component.

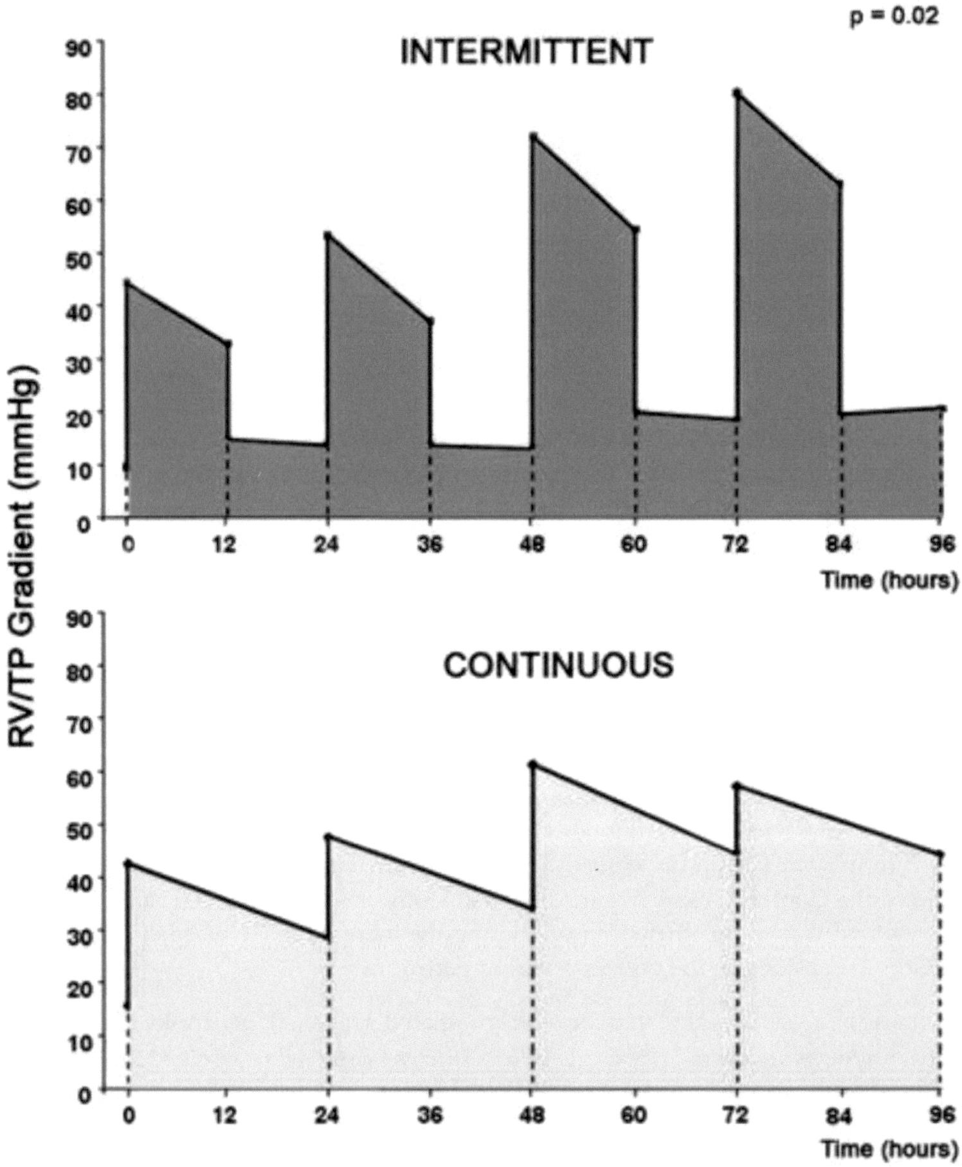

Lower graph: RV to Pulmonary trunk (PT) gradient (mmHg) of group submitted to continuous RV systolic overload (*p=0.02).

Figure 10. Diagram of RV systolic overload. Upper graph: RV to Pulmonary trunk (PT) gradient (mmHg) of the group submitted to 12-hour RV systolic overload paired with 12-hour resting period.

http://dx.doi.org/10.5772/57117

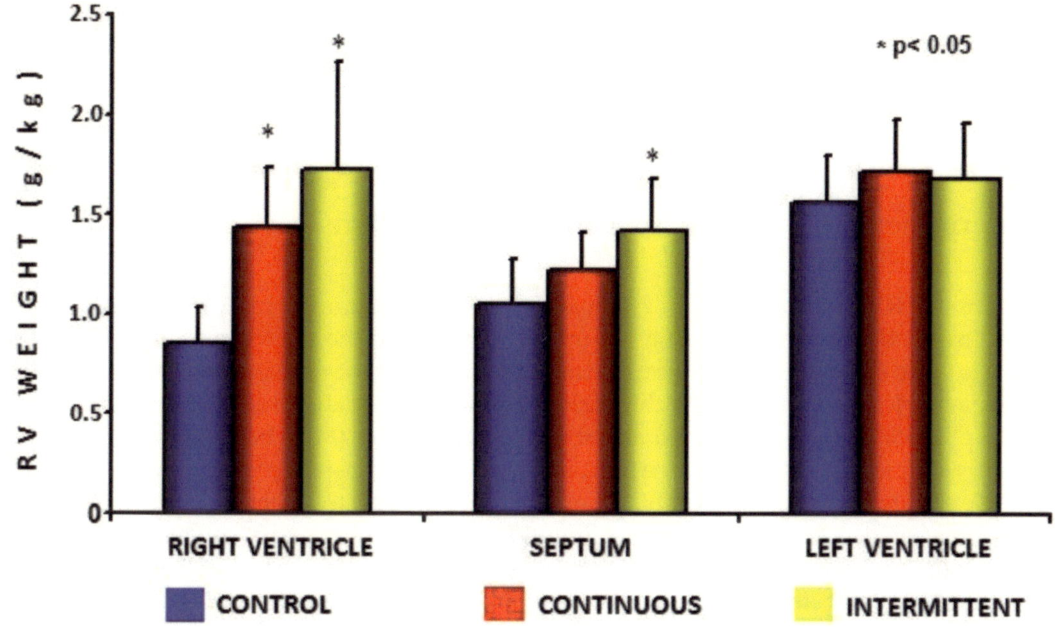

Figure 11. Cardiac masses Weight of Control, Continuous and Intermittent Groups. Similar increase in the RV masses of both stimulated groups was observed, as compared to Control Group ($p<0.05$). Only Intermittent Group had a significant increase of septal mass ($p<0.03$), when compared to Control Group. No significant changes were seen in the LV mass of the three groups ($p=0.53$).

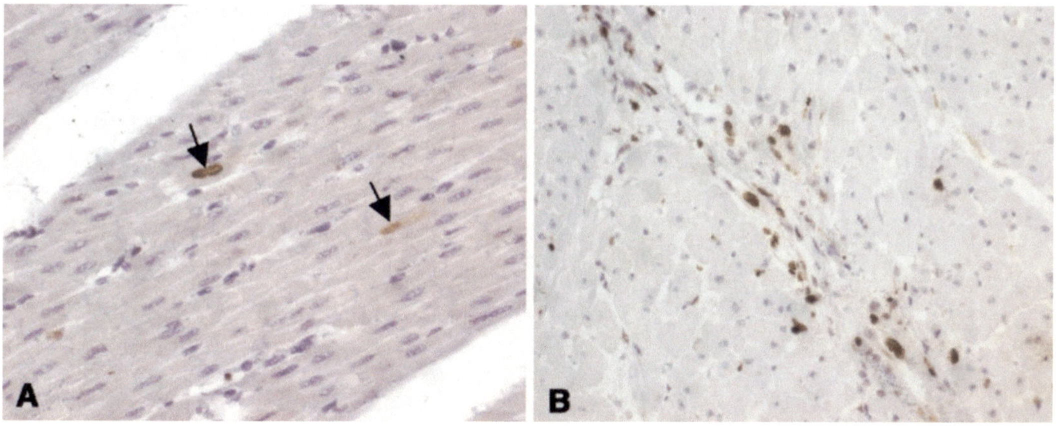

Figure 12. Histologic aspect of Ki-67-labeled cardiomyocytes. Higher indexes of proliferating cells were found in the RV of both stimulated groups (Continuous group, 1.13%; Intermittent group, 0.68%) when compared with the corresponding LV and ventricular septum.

This hypothesis is corroborated by the studies of Le Bret et al. They have demonstrated in adult animal model that only two hours per day of RV systolic overload was capable of inducing

RV hypertrophy during a period of five weeks. On the other hand, fibrosis was observed only in animals submitted to traditional PA banding protocol, when compared to intermittent group. Therefore, it seems that the duration of the training period is important as an inductor of myocardial fibrosis, responsible for late heart failure.

5. Intermittent systolic overload and heart function

Evaluation of RV function is difficult to image because of its complex morphology. Although cardiac magnetic resonance imaging is currently considered the reference technique for RV volumetry and calculation of the ejection fraction, various echocardiographic parameters can provide reliable information on RV dimensions and RV systolic and diastolic function in daily clinical practice. Therefore, the myocardial performance index (MPI) has been proposed as a relatively simple method to assess the combined systolic and diastolic performance of the right ventricle simultaneously. Focusing on a more sensitive method to detect early disturbances in ventricular function during the process of rapid RV hypertrophy, we have compared subpulmonary ventricular function of intermittent versus continuous systolic overload, using MPI and a pharmacologic stress technique. The combination of these techniques resulted in greater sensitivity in assessing ventricular function in that protocol. A new adjustable pulmonary artery banding system, made by SILIMED Inc. (Rio de Janeiro, Brazil), was implanted just beyond the pulmonar valve (Figure 13).

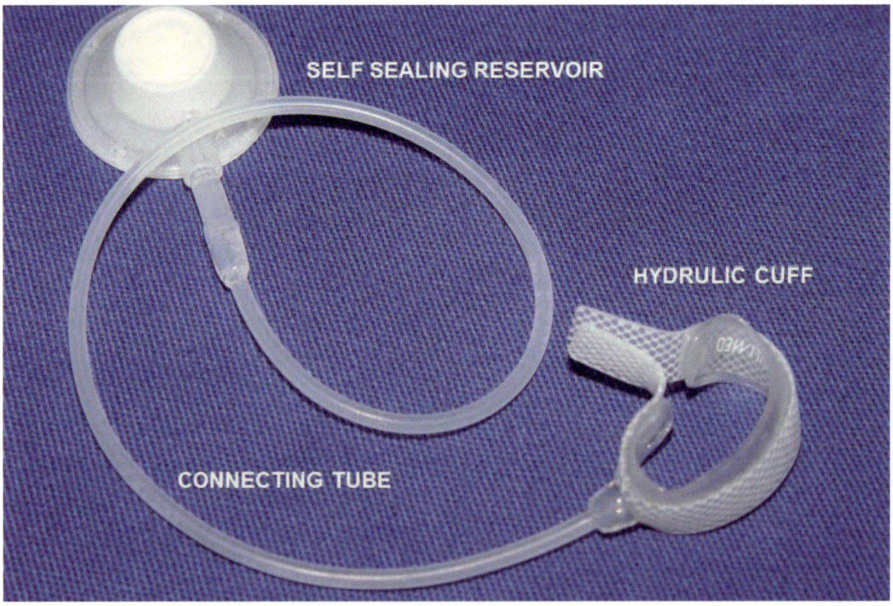

Figure 13. The adjustable pulmonary artery banding system, made by SILIMED Inc., Rio de Janeiro. The prototype has three parts: an insufflating button that includes a self-sealing silicone diaphragm at a top, a banding ring comprising a hydraulic cuff and an extending tube connecting both hermetically.

http://dx.doi.org/10.5772/57117

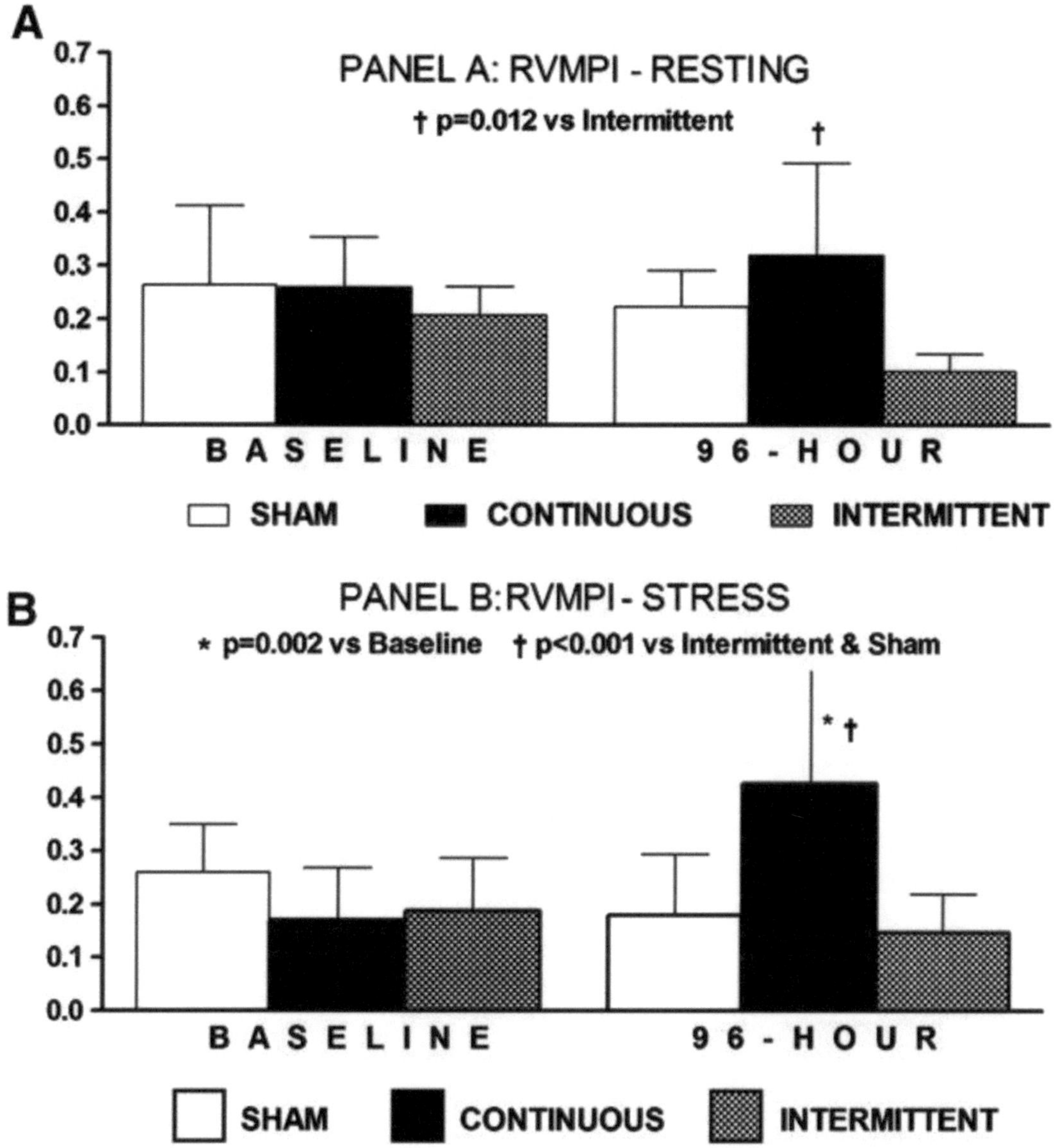

Figure 14. Right ventricular myocardial performance index (RVMPI) of sham, continuous, and intermittent groups, under dobutamine stress. A, Resting condition († p=0.012 compared with that in intermittent group at the same moment) and, B, dobutamine stress (* p=0.002 compared with baseline value; † p<0.001 compared with that in intermittent and sham groups at the same moment).

It has been demonstrated that intermittent systolic overload promoted a functionally superior hypertrophy at rest and under dobutamine stress, and that MPI enhances diagnostic confidence in ventricular retraining (Figure 14).

Regarding RV end diastolic volume, continuous systolic overload resulted in persistent dilation throughout the protocol (Figure 15). This could also reflect worse ventricular adaptation in the continuous group. On the other hand, the 12-hour resting periods of intermittent systolic overload might have optimized subendocardial coronary flow in the intermittent group, limiting the severity of systolic overload. It would probably provide a better adaptation and consequent preservation of ventricular function in the intermittent group at periods of systolic overload.

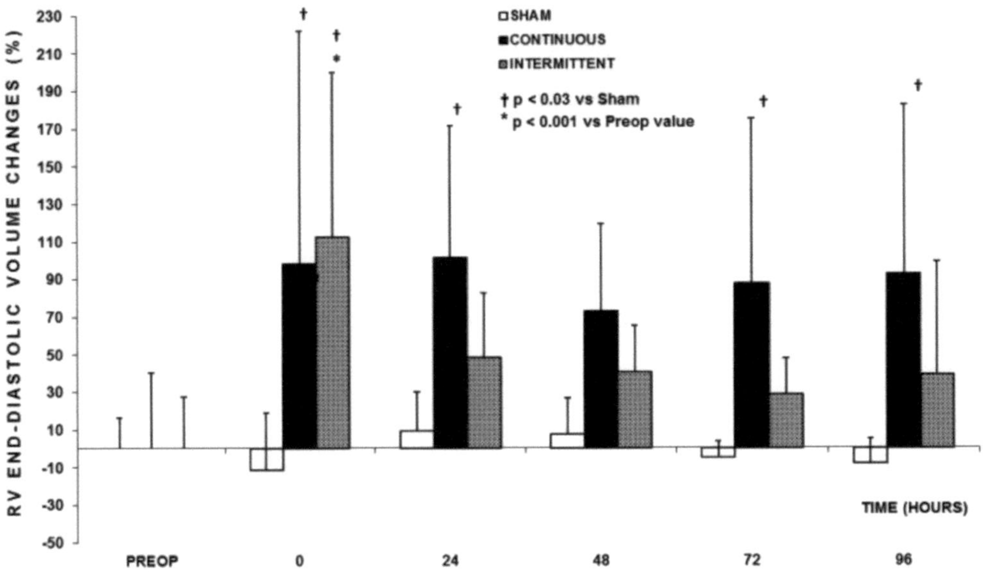

Figure 15. Right ventricular end diastolic volume changes of Sham, Continuous and Intermittent groups. † $p < 0.001$ compared with that of the sham group. * $p < 0.001$ compared with its respective baseline value.

6. Intermittent systolic overload and energetic metabolism

It is essential to understand the molecular mechanisms involved in PAB-induced myocardial hypertrophy to establish training protocols that lead to a desirable "physiologic hypertrophy" versus a deleterious "pathologic hypertrophy." Because a known shift occurs in energy substrate use in favor of glucose in pathologic conditions, energy metabolism might be altered in PAB ventricular retraining protocols. In addition, recent experimental studies have linked an unbalanced oxidative and reductive process to a variety of diseases, such as atherosclerosis and heart failure. Glucose 6-phosphate dehydrogenase (G6PD), the rate limiting enzyme that commits glucose to the pentose phosphate pathway, is mainly responsible for the generation of nicotinamide adenine dinucleotide phosphate (NADPH) and ribose 5-phosphate, an essential precursor of the de novo synthesis of RNA and DNA. G6PD-derived NADPH, a cofactor for glutathione and thioredoxin reductase, preserves reducing potentials and protects the cell from oxidative stress in normal conditions. In human diseases, G6PD can be either activated or inhibited; however, evidence has emerged that the overexpression and activation of G6PD enhances NADPH oxidase–derived superoxide generation and increases oxidative stress in diseases like diabetes, heart failure, and hypertension. In regard to rapid ventricular training, it is of great interest to evaluate myocardial energy metabolism in response to different cardiac hypertrophy models and its relationship to heart function. We have compared the myocardial G6PD activity of young goats in 2 RV training protocols, continuous versus intermittent systolic overload (Figure 16).

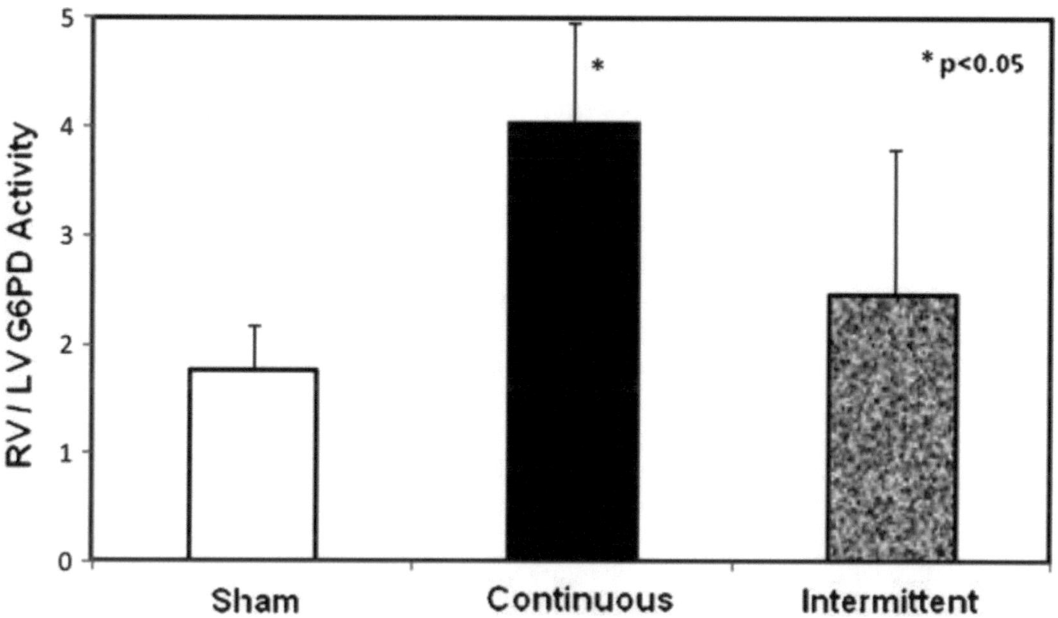

Figure 16. RV/LV ratio of G6PD activity in the sham, continuous, and intermittent groups. *p<0.05 compared with that in the sham and intermittent groups.

The continuous group presented a series of deleterious effects during rapid subpulmonary ventricle retraining. Persistent RV dilation was followed by impaired RV function and increased G6PD activity. Because the pentose phosphate pathway is one of the major sources of NADPH in cardiac myocytes, this is an important finding, and it may indicate an unbalanced redox, with the occurrence of oxidative stress and generation of reactive oxygen species related to NADPH oxidase. The final consequence of this cascade of events would be the cardiomyopathy related to protein aggregation owing to reductive stress. It has been demonstrated that either G6PD activation or inhibition is associated with diseases. However, growing evidence has emerged that G6PD overexpression correlates with oxidative and reductive stress, and new investigational drugs are currently under development to suppress its action. For instance, diabetic patients had upregulation of G6PD with high NADPH levels, and that was linked to inhibition of nitric oxide synthesis and endothelial dysfunction. Although the mechanisms underlying the increased production of reactive oxygen species in the heart are not completely understood, it has been proposed that the high rate of glucose oxidation increases mitochondrial membrane potential, which enhances production of superoxide anion. The latter would be a modulator in diabetic vasculopathy and precede the development of diabetic cardiomyopathy. We speculate that, in case of persistent systolic overload, upregulation and hyperactivity of myocardial G6PD observed in the continuous group strongly suggest that the pentose phosphate pathway enhances cytosolic NADPH availability, thus fueling free radical production by NADPH oxidase and uncoupled nitric oxide synthase. Therefore, it may induce superoxide anion myocardial injury, as well as protein aggregation, and subsequently heart failure. We postulate that intermittent systolic overload promotes the desirable effects of myocardial hypertrophy without its adverse effects. We would argue that the 12-hour resting period allowed the myocardium to replenish energy substrates and reestablish subendocardial perfusion owing to a lower ventricular wall tension. That would probably provide better hemodynamic performance at periods of systolic overload.

It is difficult to make definitive conclusions about a hypertrophic process based on a single enzyme activity. Nevertheless, it is essential to correlate these biochemical findings with production of superoxide anions and apoptosis to better understand the role of oxidative stress in hypertrophy training protocols. Previous studies have demonstrated that the oxidative branch of the pentose phosphate pathway, which produces NADPH and ribulose 5-phosphate, is essentially irreversible, being controlled primarily by G6PD activity and, hence, the NADPH/NADP ratio. NADPH oxidase preferentially uses NADPH derived from the pentose phosphate pathway, and that, in the failing heart, more glucose is oxidized through the pentose phosphate pathway, with a consequent increase in electron donors available to fuel O_2 generating enzymes. Maybe that is the way $NADP^+$ is upregulated. Although this is a non-specific pathway of free radical production, we have found a concordance of impaired RV function of continuous group and increased G6PD. Nevertheless, it would be more objective if oxygen-derived free radicals or tissue injury markers related to their production had been measured. Therefore, it is somehow difficult to assume and interpret a whole metabolic pathway based on the activity of a single enzyme. The hyperactivity in myocardial G6PD, together with RV dilation and dysfunction, may be related to an unbalanced redox determined by a constant and pathologic systolic overload. Given that pentose phosphate pathway enhances cytosolic NADPH availability, this altered energy substrate metabolism can elevate levels of free radicals by NADPH oxidase, an important mechanism in the pathophysiology of heart failure. On the other hand, intermittent systolic overload has promoted a more efficient RV hypertrophy than the continuous one, with better preservation of myocardial performance and smaller G6PD activity.

7. Mature ventricle retraining

Although the survival of patients with CCTGA is dictated largely by the associated defects, life expectancy is diminished for patients even with the isolated form of the condition. A

http://dx.doi.org/10.5772/57117

number of studies have confirmed that life expectancy is substantially diminished even for patients who have reached adulthood. The most common cause of death is congestive heart failure secondary to morphologically right (systemic) ventricular dysfunction, often associated with regurgitation of the tricuspid valve. The traditional surgical approach to the treatment of patients with CCTGA maintains the morphologically RV and tricuspid valve in the systemic circulation. However, dysfunction of the systemic (morphologically right) ventricle or systemic atrioventricular (tricuspid) valve tends to develop and worsen with time, which may lead to significant morbidity and mortality. Tricuspid regurgitation can be addressed by valvuloplasty or replacement of the systemic atrioventricular valve. Nevertheless, this procedure is often unsuccessful in preventing or reversing right ventricular dysfunction. There are indeed anatomical and physiological considerations that support the assumption that the LV is more suitable than the right to serve the systemic circulation. First of all, LV (with its cylindrical shape, its concentric contraction pattern, and both the inlet and outlet orifices situated in close proximity) seems ideally adapted to work as a pressure pump, whereas the RV (with its crescent-shaped cavity, its large internal surface area-to-volume ratio, its bellows-like contraction pattern, and its more separated inlet and outlet segments) seems better suited to serve as a low-pressure volume pump chamber. Also, the LV has two coronary arteries (left anterior descending and circumflex), while the RV has only one (right coronary). Furthermore, the papillary muscles of the RV are small and numerous, originating both from the septum and from the right ventricular free wall, in contrast to the two papillary muscles of the LV. This architecture allows the tricuspid valve to be pulled apart as the RV dilates, leading to tricuspid regurgitation. In long-term, patients with CCTGA begins to dilate RV and the tricuspid annulus (which is the systemic valve), allowing RV blood regurgitation during ventricular contraction and, consequently, pulmonary congestion and dyspnea. The high late mortality associated with the traditional approach has stimulated a number of groups to propose a more anatomic repair on the basis of the hypothesis that establishment of atrioventricular and ventriculoarterial concordance would improve the long term survival of patients with this anomaly. This approach has been named as double switch operation, i.e., atrial level circulation switch by the Senning procedure and arterial switch operation at the same time. This strategy has the appealing theoretic advantage of recruiting the morphologically LV and mitral valve to sustain systemic pressure and resistance, thus relieving the hemodynamic burden on the RV and tricuspid valve. Many of these patients are older and are seen because of right ventricular failure, usually with tricuspid valve regurgitation and often without associated defects. As would be expected in these cases, the LV is physiologically unprepared to sustain systemic pressure and resistance, because it has been working as the pulmonary ventricle. Therefore, double switch procedure must be performed after a preliminary PA banding procedure to recondition the LV. Although PAB appears to be capable of providing adequate LV training when done at an early age, it is not always suitable for mature myocardium, with disappointing results in older patients. Because of the high degree of variability among these patients, optimal band tightness is not always achieved on the first effort and is often limited by the onset of LV dysfunction. The retraining process of the LV, especially in older patients, may take months before obtaining the necessary LV hypertrophy to sustain systemic pressure and vascular resistance. According to Mavroudis and Backer, in patients with TGA and failed atrial inversion, aged from 1.9 to 23 years, it took an average of 15.6 months to retrain the subpulmonary ventricle for the two-stage Jatene operation. In addition, it has been described in the literature the need for subsequent reoperations to readjust PA banding in cases where patient cannot achieve adequate LV hypertrophy. The difficulties in retraining adult myocardium with the traditional approach has stimulated several groups to propose a more physiologic protocol based on the hypothesis that intermittent systolic overload would improve the quality of subpulmonary ventricle hypertrophy. Such an approach has the appealing advantage of ventricular retraining with no collagen formation, providing a more physiologic hypertrophy. However, the time necessary to retrain these ventricles and the best way to achieve a more physiologic hypertrophy and assess the specific histologic changes involved in this process are still required. We have compared the histomorphometric changes of PAB-induced RV hypertrophy of adult goats, with the emphasis on a detailed analysis of the myocardium adaptation process (Table 1).

	Sham N = 6	**Traditional** N = 6	**Intermmitent** N = 6	**p value**
Mass (g/kg)	0.79 ± 0.15	1.08 ± 0.17 *	1,24 ± 0.16 †	<0.05
Water Content (%)	79.16 ± 1.28	79.67 ± 1.25	80.61 ± 1.87	0.27
Cardiomyocyte diameter (μm)	11.54 ± 0.89	12.96 ± 1.35	13.76 ± 1.68 †	<0.05
Nuclei diameter (μm)	3.86 ± 0.14	4.40 ± 0.48	4.74 ± 0.71 †	<0.05
Collagen percentage area (%)	2.94 ± 0.65	5.82 ± 1.91 *	3.44 ± 1.24 #	<0.05
Cardiomyocyte Ki67+ cells (cells/ field)	0.33 (0.08-0.75)	0.33 (0.08-0.83)	0.25 (0.08-0.58)	0.89
Interstitial/Vessel Ki67+ cells (cells/field)	2.67 (1.00-3.58)	2.83 (1.25-8.50)	2.17 (1.75-4.75)	0.68

Values: means ± SD or medians (limits)

* p<0.05 compared Traditional and Sham groups;

† p<0.05 compared Intermittent and Sham groups;

# p<0.05 compared Intermittent and Traditional groups.

Table 1. Gross and histomorphometric RV findings in Sham, Traditional and Intermittent groups

The prototype used in this study (SILIMED, Rio de Janeiro, Brazil) represents the adult version of the small adjustable PAB system used previously in young animals (Figure 17). Its dimensions were planned to support higher pressure gradients in adolescents and adults patients considered for subpulmonary ventricle retraining. All parts of the Adjustable Banding System are made of biologically stable material (medical grade silicone).

The banding ring is a C-shaped hydraulic cuff that has three layers. The inner wall of the banding ring is formed by a very thin and flexible silicone that allows centripetal distension. Differently from the young animal prototype, the outer layer is divided in two parts, both

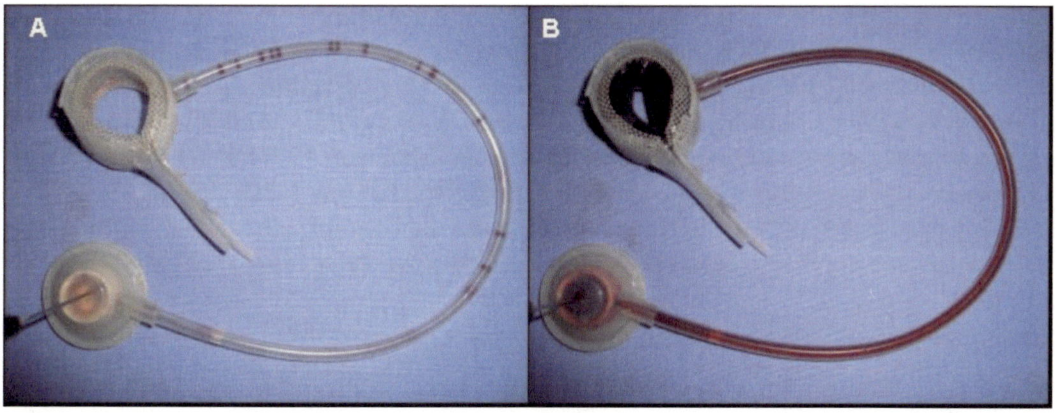

Figure 17. The adult banding device consists of an inflatable C-shaped hydraulic cuff (24-mm diameter) and an inflation reservoir connected hermetically to each other by a 2.0-mm diameter tube (SILIMED, Rio de Janeiro, Brazil).

consisting of 1.0-mm-thick rigid silicone each, reinforced with a polyester mesh. The outer external layer presents some small holes along the non apart borders, which are used for securing it firmly with sutures to the adventitia of the artery. This keeps the adjustable banding system from migrating distally and impinging on the pulmonary artery bifurcation. The external layer prolongs with two apart ends, planned for further adjustment of the hydraulic cuff, when placed around the artery, by suturing together the ends. The inner external layer prolongs alongside the cuff as a canoe, to keep it from deforming. The connecting tubing has 1.0 mm inner diameter. The inflation reservoir used to pump fluid to the hydraulic cuff consists of a ceramic cylindrical reservoir, with a self-sealing silicone diaphragm at the top, which keeps the banding system leak proof after repeated needle puncture of the reservoir.

The two regimens of ventricular training, traditional and intermittent, have promoted different degrees of myocardial hypertrophy. However, it was less intense and longer in adult animals than that observed previously in young goat hearts. Histomorphometric and echocardiographic data indicated that intermittent RV systolic overload promoted a harmless RV hypertrophy in adult goats during a 4-week study period. On one hand, the primary mechanism of RV mass acquisition was probably related to increased protein synthesis and cell hypertrophy rather than myocardial hyperplasia or edema. On the other hand, the traditional PAB group evolved with greater collagen production, which is one of the important mechanisms of late ventricular failure. The absence of myocardial edema and significant cell proliferation observed in that study suggests that the mass acquisition was probably related to enhanced protein synthesis, both intracellular (contractile proteins) and extracellular (matrix proteins). In the adult heart of mammals, it is generally believed that almost none of the cardiomyocytes proliferate and that the hypertrophy process functions as the fundamental adaptive response. The magnitude of cardiomyocyte hypertrophy then depends on the age at which the stimulus is produced. As predicted in an adult model, no significant cellular proliferation was observed in any cardiac segment, contrary to the findings of similar experimental studies in young animals, in which RV responds not only with hypertrophy of the myocardial fibers but also with hyperplasia of the contractile and interstitial myocardial cells.

Although the intermittent group was the one least exposed to systolic overload, a more efficient RV hypertrophy was observed, just as documented previously by our studies in young goat hearts. Similarly, the hemodynamic results showed that the intermittent group could achieve greater RV-to-PA pressure gradients than the traditional group during the 4-week study period. Intermittent systolic overload mimics exercise training, which can benefit the trained myocardium with improved subendocardial perfusion. On one hand, it is likely that the mechanism of this hypertrophic process may be developed during the resting periods with ideal oxygen transport and, hence, without the collagen deposition resulting from continuous

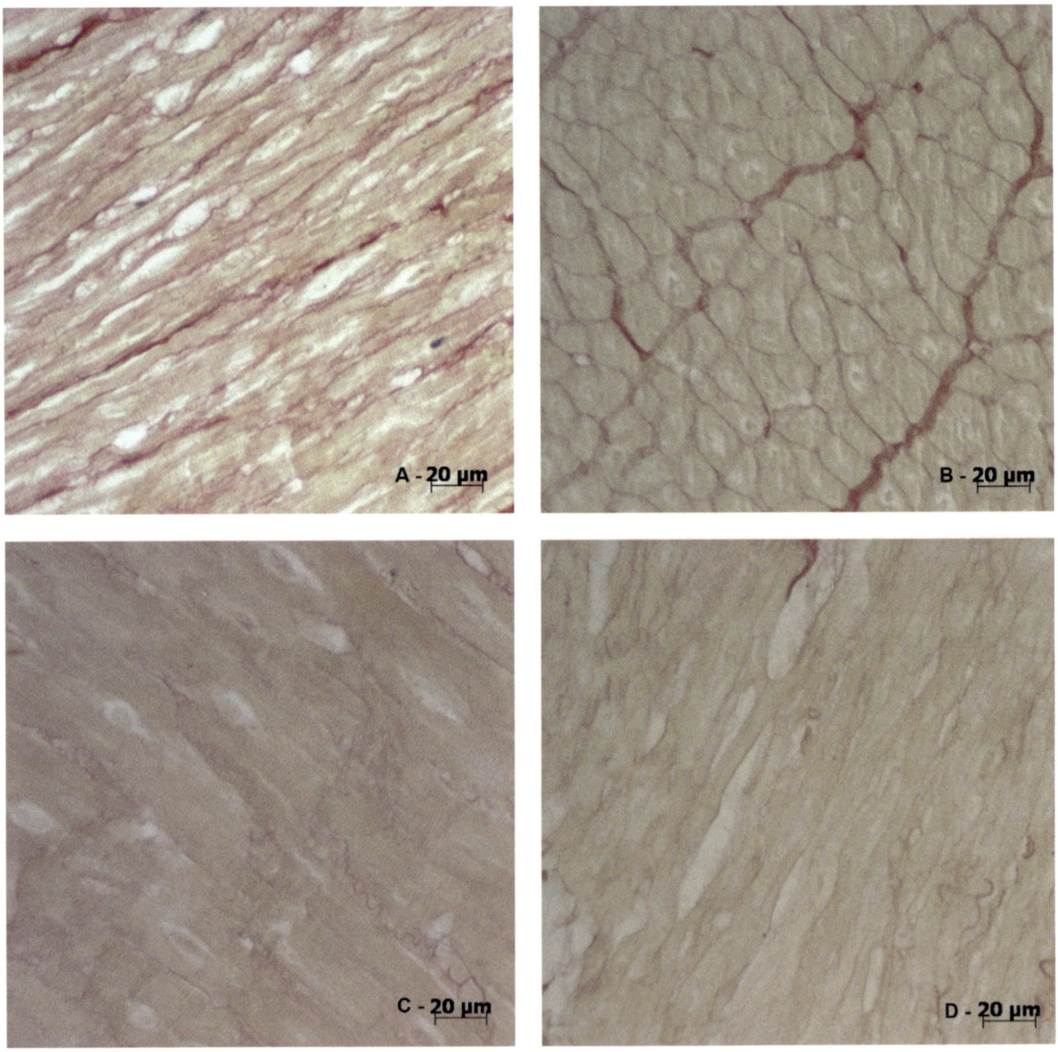

Figure 18. Photomicrographies of the right ventricular myocardium from four representative animals, two from the Traditional (A and B) and two from the Intermittent (C and D) group, after four weeks of systolic overload. Panels A and B show a higher density and intensity of collagen staining (red fibers around individual cardiomyocytes- endomysial fibrosis) than that in panels C and D. Sirius-red staining, objective magnification-20X.

http://dx.doi.org/10.5772/57117

relative diastolic hypoperfusion. On the other hand, the traditional group had deleterious effects at the end of the protocol, with more collagen deposition in the RV interstitium. The mean RV collagen area fraction of the Traditional group was significantly greater than in the Sham group (98% increase; $p<0.01$), and greater than that in the Intermittent group (69.2% increase; $p<0.05$). The histological distribution of collagen in representative animals from trained groups is demonstrated in Figure 18. This collagen deposit may be the key determinant of the impaired RV function previously observed on the same protocol. Accordingly, Le Bret and colleagues reported myocardial fibrosis associated with continuous overload and no fibrosis in their "fitness" group, during a 5-week period in adult sheep. Although the results with adjustable intermittent PAB are encouraging, it is premature to assume this as the definitive solution for adult myocardium retraining.

8. Adjustable PA banding and hypoplastic left heart syndrome

More recently, bilateral PA banding has been applied to hypoplastic left heart syndrome (HLHS). The mitral and aortic valves present either with atresia or hypoplasia. This results in a situation where the left side of the heart is completely unable to support systemic circulation, though the right side of the heart is typically normally developed. Blood returning from the lungs to the LA must pass through an atrial septal defect to the right side of the heart. The RV must then pump blood both to the lungs (via the pulmonary trunk) and out to the body (via a patent ductus arteriosus). The patent *Ductus Arteriosus*, a normal structure in the fetus, is often the only pathway through which blood can reach the body from the heart. When the *Ductus Arteriosus* begins to close, as it typically does in the first days of life, the blood flow to the body will severely diminish, resulting in dangerously low blood flow to vital organs and leading to shock. Without treatment, HLHS is uniformly fatal, often within the first hours or days of life. The most commonly pursued treatment for HLHS is "staged reconstruction" in which a series of operations, usually three, are performed to reconfigure the child's cardio-vascular system to be as efficient as possible, despite the lack of an adequate LV. The first operation in the staged approach is the Norwood operation and is typically performed in the first week of life. With the Norwood operation, the RV becomes the systemic or main ventricle pumping to the body, and a systemic-to-pulmonary shunt aims redirectioning circulatory pathways to protect the pulmonary vasculature from excessive blood flow and optimize systemic organ flows. However, some overloading of the systemic right ventricle still persists after this operation. Also, such major surgical procedure is usually performed in the neonatal period (sometimes in a low-birth weight patient and unfavorable anatomy), which may result in sub-optimal neurological outcomes in the long-term. Because of the extensive reconstruction of the aorta that must be done, this operation is one of the most challenging heart surgeries in Pediatrics. This traditional surgical approach of newborns with HLHS is complex and continues to have significant mortality compared with other neonatal cardiac operations.

An alternative approach for palliation of hypoplastic left heart in the neonatal period has been stenting the arterial duct in combination with branch PA banding and atrial septostomy, as needed. The so called hybrid stage I palliation has been considered the preferred therapeutic approach in high-risk neonates. However, fine adjustments of the amount of pulmonary blood flow, which is a critical issue, has proved to be a particularly difficult aspect of the procedure. This can be readily explained when it is recalled that Poiseuille's law predicts that blood flow is related to the fourth power of the radius of the vessel. Therefore, a minor alteration in diameter will have a large impact on flow and pressure gradient across the band site. Generally, the bands are surgically adjusted (tighten or loosened), based on pressure measurements and the arterial oxygen saturation monitoring. A systolic pressure in the distal pulmonary artery less than half of the systemic pressure and an arterial oxygen saturation of 75%-85% usually reflect an adequate balance between the pulmonary and systemic blood flow. This may be readily achieved in the operating room, with an open chest and under artificial conditions. However, in the postoperative period, which may be quite unpredictable, the fixed pulmonary bandings do not allow for fine adjustments according to the underlying clinical needs of the patient. Moreover, in order to avoid hypoxemia as the infant rapidly grows up, the balance between the pulmonary and systemic blood flows should be adjusted, which is impossible with the fixed bands. To deal with these problems, we devised a mini banding device that allows for fine percutaneous adjustments of the pulmonary blood flow in the neonate (Figure 19). The banding ring is a C-shaped hydraulic cuff, with 5 mm width, and a rigid outer layer, reinforced with a polyester mesh, which keep it from deforming centrifugally. It can be used in pulmonary arteries varying from 3 mm to 6 mm internal diameter range.

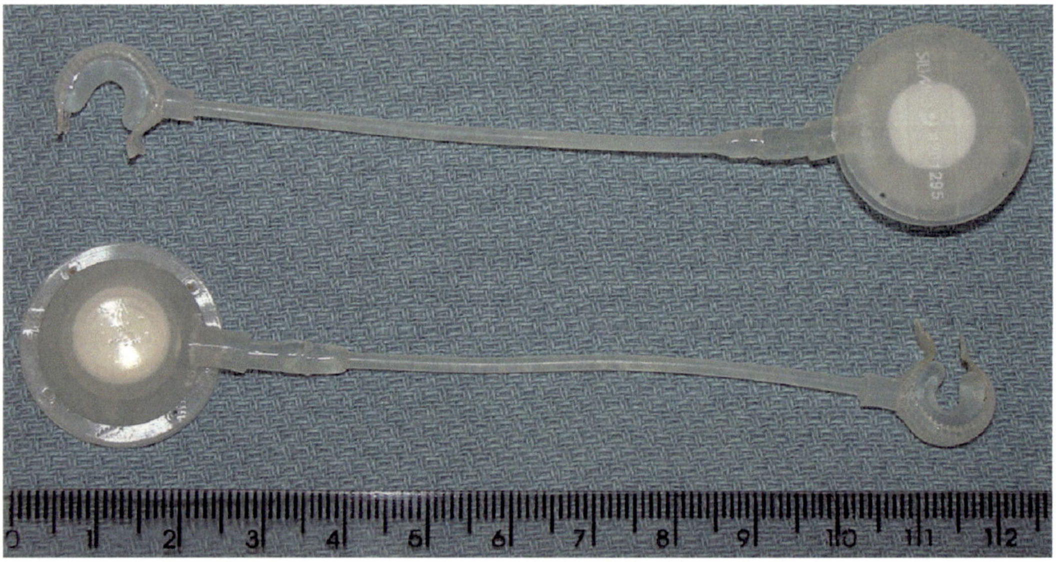

Figure 19. The adjustable pulmonary artery banding system (SILIMED, Rio de Janeiro, Brazil) used for Hybrid Stage I palliation for HLHS.

This innovative percutaneous mini adjustable banding system permits a fine control of the pulmonary blood flow by increasing or decreasing accurately the cross-sectional diameter of the pulmonary arteries. Therefore, it is adjusted according to the underlying clinical conditions of the patients: hypoxemia is, for instance, managed by unfastening the pulmonary artery banding circumference. Once the adjustable banding ring is placed around the PA's and the inflation reservoirs left in the infraclavicular subcutaneous tissue, the degree of banding rings constriction is adjusted after sternal closure (Figure 20). Each band is inflated with saline solution to decrease arterial oxygen saturation to the 75%-85% range, while breathing under a 30% inspired oxygen fraction.

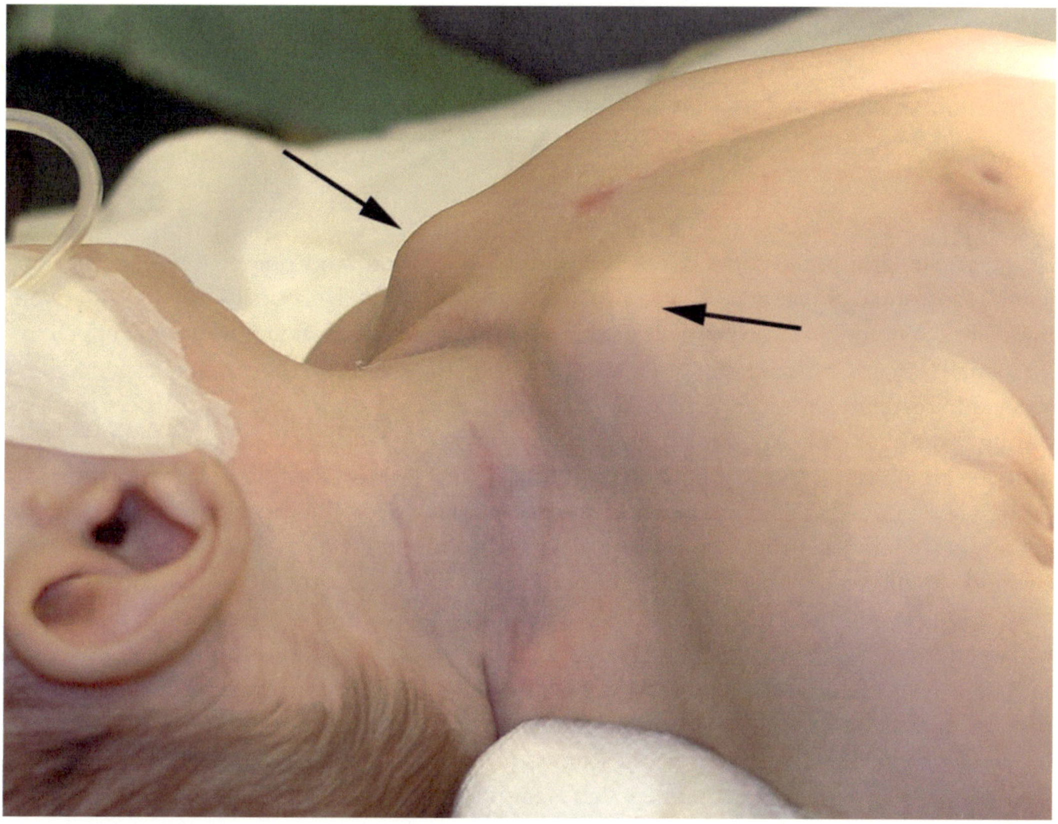

Figure 20. Inflating reservoirs positioned in the infraclavicular area (arrows), one for each pulmonary artery for independent percutaneous blood flow adjustment.

We have performed Hybrid Stage I palliation for HLHS using the adjustable PA band (APAB group) in 3 patients (1.8 kg - 2.8 kg) and traditional bands (TPAB group) in 3 patients (2.0 kg - 3.3 kg). The babies were followed closely with serial echocardiographic assessment every week. During inter-stage 1-2, several additional percutaneous adjustments of the PA's banding systems were necessary to maintain the arterial oxygen saturation in the recommended range according to somatic growth. Figure 21 shows the O_2 saturation behavior of both groups during interstage 1-2 period.

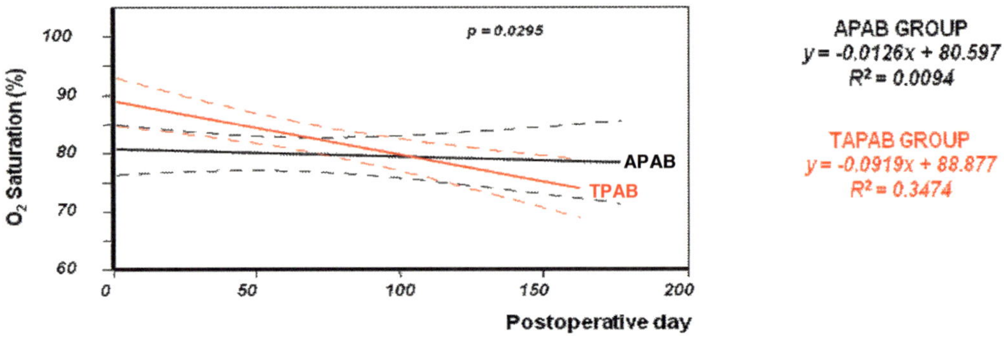

Figure 21. Traditional PA banding group evolved with progressive decrease of oxygen saturation during interstage 1-2, while the group using adjustable PA bands maintained more stable arterial oxygen saturation according to somatic growth.

In the APAB group, all patients reached stage 2 operation, and one of them has already completed Fontan circulation at 2 years of age, while in the TPAB group, two cases underwent the stage 2 operation and one patient died just before stage 2 operation (pulmonary infection). This small series of HLHS cases demonstrated that customization of the pulmonary blood flow seemed to result in a more precise balance between the pulmonary and systemic circulations during the interstage 1-2 period. The use of adjustable PA bands in the stage-1 hybrid procedure for HLHS can provide a more stable clinical condition, according to the rapid somatic growth and underlying clinical needs of the patient. However, the calibration of the banding cuffs was sometimes difficult to achieve, due to the extreme complexity of the continuously changing relationship between systemic and pulmonary vascular resistance, with the dependency upon several inter-related variable such as the values of the arterial pO2, pCO2, pH, hemoglobin, cardiac output, level of sedation, use of peripheral and/or pulmonary vasodilators, etc. Nevertheless, fine and reversible adjustments could be performed as many times as needed, both in acute and ambulatory settings, avoiding further surgical interventions. The use of this innovative banding system seemed to result in a more predictable postoperative course, and in a more stable patient, which is highly desirable for the comprehensive phase II operation. A concern with any PAB technique or device, including ours, is the possibility of causing vessel distortions or stenoses, which may have a deleterious impact for subsequent cavo-pulmonary operations. Fortunately, the scar tissue surrounding the banding devices was minimal in our patient and did not result in any of these complications. The cases electively submitted to the "comprehensive" stage II surgical palliation showed the anatomy of the pulmonary arteries well preserved with no distortions.

In summary, the use of our innovative mini PAB system allowed for a fine control of the pulmonary blood flow in neonates with HLHS undergoing phase I palliation. This customization of the pulmonary blood flow according to the underlying clinical needs of an infant with rapid somatic growth seemed to result in a more precise balance between the pulmonary and systemic circulations during the inter-stage period.

http://dx.doi.org/10.5772/57117

Author details

Renato S. Assad

Heart Institute University of Sao Paulo School of Medicine, Brazil

References

[1] Bishop SP & Cole CR – Production of Externally Controlled Progressive Pulmonis Stenosis in the Dog. J Appl Physiol. 1969; 26:659-63.

[2] Assad RS, Cardarelli M, Abduch MCD, Aiello VD, Maizato M, Jatene A.D. Bandagem Reversível do Tronco Pulmonar: Modelo Experimental para Preparo Rápido do Ventrículo Pulmonar. Rev Bras Cir Cardiovasc. 1998; 13: 239-48.

[3] Jacobson JH & McAllister FF. A method for the controlled occlusion of a larger blood vessels. Ann Surg. 1957; 145:334-43.

[4] Edmunds LHJr, Rudy LW, Heymann MA, Boucher JK. An adjustable pulmonary arterial band. Trans Am Soc Artif Int Organs. 1972; 18:217-25.

[5] Park SC, Griffith BP, Siewers RD, Hardesty RL, Ladowsky J, Zoltum RA, Neches WH, Zuberbuhler JR. A percutaneously adjustable device for banding of the pulmonary trunk. Int J Cardiol. 1985; 9:477-84.

[6] Solis E, Heck CF, Seward JB, Kaye MP. Percutaneously adjustable pulmonary artery band. Ann Thorac Surg. 1986; 41:65-9.

[7] Jonas RA, Giglia TM, Sanders SP, Wernovsky G, Nadal-Ginard B, Mayer JE Jr, Castaneda AR. Rapid Two-Stage Arterial Switch for Transposition of the Great Arteries and Intact Ventricular Septum beyond the Neonatal Period. Circulation. 1989; 80: I203-8.

[8] Yacoub MH, Radley-Smith R, Maclaurin R: Two-stage operation for anatomical correction of transposition of the great arteries with intact interventricular septum. Lancet. 1977;1: 1275-8.

[9] Mee RB. Severe right ventricular failure after Mustard or Senning operation. Two-stage repair: pulmonary artery banding and switch. J Thorac Cardiovasc Surg. 1986;92:385-90.

[10] Mavroudis C, Backer CL. Arterial switch after failed atrial baffle procedures for transposition of the great arteries. Ann Thorac Surg. 2000; 69:851-857.

[11] van Son JA, Reddy VM, Silverman NH, Hanley FL. Regression of tricuspid regurgitation after two-stage arterial switch operation for failing systemic ventricle after atrial inversion operation. J Thorac Cardiovasc Surg. 1996; 111: 342-7.

[12] Devaney EJ, Ohye RG, Bove EL. Technical aspects of the combined arterial switch and senning operation for congenitally corrected transposition of the great arteries. Semin Thorac Cardiovasc Surg Pediatr Card Surg Annu. 2003;6:9-15.

[13] Devaney EJ, Charpie JR, Ohye RG, Bove EL. Combined arterial switch and Senning operation for congenitally corrected transposition of the great arteries: patient selection and intermediate results. J Thorac Cardiovasc Surg. 2003;125: 500-7.

[14] Mee RB. The double switch operation with accent on the Senning component. Semin Thorac Cardiovasc Surg Pediatr Card Surg Annu. 2005:57-65.

[15] Winlaw DS, McGuirk SP, Balmer C. Intention-to-treat analysis of pulmonary artery banding in conditions with a morphological right ventricle in the systemic circulation with a view to anatomic biventricular repair. Circulation. 2005; 111: 405-11.

[16] Duncan BW, Mee RB, Mesia CI, Qureshi A, Rosenthal GL, Seshadri SG, Lane GK, Latson LA. Results of the double switch operation for congenitally corrected transposition of the great arteries. Eur J Cardiothorac Surg. 2003; 24: 11-9; discussion 19-20.

[17] Sidi D, Heurtematte Y, kachaner J, Fermont L, Batisse E, Villain A, Hazan E, Lecompte Y. Problems posed by preparation of the left ventricle for anatomical correction in simple transposition of the great vessels. Arch Mal Coeur Vaiss. 1983. 76:575-83.

[18] Colan SD, Boutin C, Castaneda AR, Wernovsky G. Status of the left ventricle after arterial switch operation for transposition of the great arteries. Hemodynamic and echocardiographic evaluation. J Thorac Cardiovasc Surg. 1955; 109:311-21.

[19] Sadoshima J, Izumo S. The celular and molecular response of cardiac myocytes to mechanical stress. Annu Rev Physiol. 1997; 59:551-71.

[20] Homcy CJ. Signaling hypertrophy: how many switches, how many wires. Circulation. 1998; 97:1890-2.

[21] Izumo S, Nadal-Guinard B, Mahdavi V. Proto-oncogene induction and reprogramming of cardiac gene expression produced by pressure overload. Proc Natl. Acad. Sci. U.S.A., 1988; 85:339-43.

[22] Rozich JD, Barnes MA, Schmid PG, Zile MR, Mcdermott PJ. Cooper 4th, G. Load effects on gene expression during cardiac hypertrophy. J Mol Cell Cardiol. 1995; 27:485-99.

[23] Boutin C, Wernovsky G, Sanders SP, Jonas RA, Castañeda A, Colan SD. Rapid two-stage arterial switch operation: evaluation of left ventricular systolic mechanics late after in acute pressure overload stimulus in infancy. Circulation. 1994; 90: 1294-303.

[24] Bishop SP, Melsen LR. Myocardial necrosis, fibrosis, and DNA synthesis in experimental cardiac hypertrophy induced by sudden pressure overload. Circ Res. 1976; 39: 238-45.

[25] Weber KT, Janicki JS, Pick R, Abrahams C, Shroff SG, Bashey RI, Chen RM. Collagen in the hypertrophied, pressure-overloaded myocardium Circulation. 1987; 75 : I 40-7.

[26] Takahashi Y, Nakano S, Shimazaki Y, Kadoba K, Taniguchi K, Sano T, Nakada T, Tsuchitani Y, Miyamoto K, Matsuda H. Echocardiographic comparison of postoperative left ventricular contractile state between one and two-stage arterial switch operation for simple transposition of the great arteries. Circulation. 1991; 84: III-180.

[27] Rabello RR, Assad RS, Krieger JE, Abduch MC, Oliveira SA. Evaluation of angiotensin converting enzyme activity in acute right ventricular hypertrophy in an experimental model of adjustable endovascular stenosis of the pulmonary trunk. Rev Bras Cir Cardiovasc. 2001; 16: 364-75.

[28] Assad RS, Rodriguez MAQ, Abduch MCD, Valente AS, Andrade JL, Krieger JE, Barbero-Marcial ML. Adjustable pulmonary trunk banding: comparison of two methods of acute subpulmonary ventricle hypertrophy. Rev Bras Cir Cardiovasc. 2006; 21: 418-428.

[29] Le Bret E, Lupoglazoff JM, Borenstein N, Fromont G, Laborde F, Bachet J, Vouhe P. Cardiac "fitness" training: an experimental comparative study of three methods of pulmonary artery banding for ventricular training. Ann Thorac Surg. 2005;79:198-203.

[30] Dias CA, Assad RS, Câneo LF, Abduch MC, Aiello VD, Dias AR, Marcial MB, Oliveira SA. Reversible Pulmonary Trunk Banding II: An Experimental Model for Rapid Pulmonary Ventricle Hypertrophy. J Thorac Cardiovasc Surg. 2002; 124:999-1006.

[31] Câneo LF, Dias CA, Assad RS, Abduch MCD, Aiello VD, Pinho Moreira LF, Lourenço- Filho D, Stolf NAG. Preparation of the pulmonary ventricle using two adjustable devices for pulmonary trunk banding. Rev Bras Cir Cardiovasc. 2001; 16: 35-48.

[32] Boutin C, Jonas RA, Sanders SP, Wernovsky G, Mone SM, Colan SD. Rapid two-stage arterial switch operation. Acquisition of left ventricular mass after pulmonary artery banding in infants with transposition of the great arteries. Circulation. 1994; 90:1304-09

[33] Yacoub M, Bernhard A, Lange P, Radley-Smith R, Keck E, Stephan E, Heintzen P : Clinical and Hemodynamic Results of the Two-stage Anatomic Correction of Simple Transposition of the Great Arteries. Circulation 1980; 62(suppl I):190-196

[34] Yasui H, Kado H, Yonenaga K, Hisahara M, Ando H, Iwao H, Fukuda S, Mizoguchi Y, Sunagawa H: arterial switch operation for transpositions of the great arteries, with special reference to left ventricular function. J Thorac Cardiovasc Surg. 1989;98:601-610

[35] Borow KM, Arensman FW, Webb C, Radley-Smith R, Yacoub MH: Assessment of left ventricular contractile state after anatomic correction of transposition of great arteries.Circulation. 1984;69:106-112

[36] Bonhoeeffer P, Henry GW, Katanhama H. Preparation of the "pulmonary ventricle" for arterial switch by adjustable intravascular ballon outflow obstruction: an experimental approach in a lamb model. Cardiol. Young. 1992;2:85-88

[37] Bonhoeeffer P, Carminati M, Parenzan L, Tynam M. Non-surgical left ventricular preparation for arterial switch in transposition of the great arteries. Lancet. 1992;340:549-550

[38] Katayama H, Krzeski R, Frantz EG, Ferrero JI, Lucas CL, Há B, Henry GW. Induction of right ventricular hypertrophy with obstructiong balloon catheter. Non-surgical ventricular preparation for the arterial switch operation in simple ransposition. Circulation. 1993;88(4 Pt 1):1765-1769

[39] Bonnet D, Maillard A, Chetboul V, Pouchelon JL, Aggoun Y, Acar P, Kachaner J, Sidi D, Bonhoeffer P. Préparation non chirurgicaledu ventricle sous-pulmonaire à la détransposition artérielle: mise au point d'um modèle animal chez l'agneau. Arch Mal Coeur Vaiss. 1997;90 :707-712

[40] Krzeski R, Katayama H, Bonhoeffer P, Lucas CL, Long WA, Parezan L, Henry GW. Obstructing ballon catheter for the induction of systolic hypertension in the pulmonary ventricle – an acute hemodynamic study in the piglet. Cardiol Young. 1992;2:89-94

[41] Mee RBB. Arterial switch for right ventricular failure following Mustard or Senning operation. In: Stark J, Pacifico A, eds. Reoperations in Cardiac Surgery. Heidelberg:Springer,1989; 217-232.

[42] Perrino C, Prasad SV, Mao L, Noma T, Yan Z, Kim HS, Smithies O, Rockman HA. Intermittent pressure overload triggers hypertrophy-independent cardiac dysfunction and vascular rarefaction. J Clin Invest. 2006;116:1547-1560.

[43] Abduch MC, Assad RS, Rodriguez MQ, Valente AS, Andrade JL, Demarchi LM, Marcial MB, Aiello VD. Reversible pulmonary trunk banding III: assessment of myocardial adaptive mechanisms-contribution of cell proliferation. J Thorac Cardiovasc Surg. 2007;133:1510-6.

[44] Miana LA, Assad RS, Abduch MC, Gomes GS, Nogueira AR, Oliveira FS, Telles BL, Souto MT, Silva GJ, Stolf NA. Intermittent systolic overload promotes better myocardial performance in adult animals. Arq Bras Cardiol. 2010;95(3):364-72.

[45] Assad RS, Atik FA, Oliveira FS, Fonseca-Alaniz MH, Abduch MC, Silva GJ, Favaro GG, Krieger JE, Stolf NA. Reversible pulmonary trunk banding. VI: Glucose-6-phosphate dehydrogenase activity in rapid ventricular hypertrophy in young goats. J Thorac Cardiovasc Surg. 2011;142:1108-13.

[46] Valente AS, Assad RS, Abduch MC, Silva GJ, Thomaz PG, Miana LA, Krieger JE, Stolf NA. Reversible pulmonary trunk banding. IV: analysis of right ventricle acute

hypertrophy in an intermittent systolic overload model. Braz J Cardiovasc Surg. 2008; 23:60-9.

[47] Carroll SM, Nimmo LE, Knoepfler PS, White FC, Bloor CM. Gene expression in a swine model of right ventricular hypertrophy: intracellular adhesion molecule, vascular endothelial growth factor and plasminogen activators are upregulated during pressure overload. J Mol Cell Cardiol.1995;27:1427-41.

[48] Leeuwenburgh BP, Steendijk P, Helbing WA, Baan J. Indexes of diastolic RV function: load dependence and changes after chronic RV pressure overload in lambs. Am J Physiol Heart Circ Physiol.2002;282(4):1350-8.

[49] Kang N, de Leval MR, Elliot M, Tsang V, Kocyildirim E, Sehic I, Foran J, Sullivan I. Extending the boundaries of the primary arterial switch operation in patients with transposition of the great arteries and intact ventricular septum. Circulation. 2004;110:123-7.

[50] Lacour GF, Piot D, Zoghbi J, Serraf A, Gruber P, Macé L, et al. Surgical management and indication of left ventricular retraining in arterial switch for transposition of great arteries with intact ventricular septum. Eur J Cardiothorac Surg.2001;20 (4): 824-9.

[51] Parker NM, Zuhdi M, Kouatli A, Baslaim G. Late presenters with dextro-transposition of great arteries and intact ventricular septum: to train or not to train the left ventricle for arterial switch operation. Congenit Heart Dis.2009;4(6):424-32.

[52] Bisoi AK, Sharma P, Chauhan S, Reddy SM, Das S, Saxena A, Kothari SS. Primary arterial switch operation in children presenting late with d-transposition of great arteries and intact ventricular septum. ′When is it too late for a primary arterial switch operation? Eur J Cardiothorac Surg. 2010;38:707-713.

[53] Edwin F, Mamorare H, Brink J, Kinsley R. Primary arterial switch operation for transposition of the great arteries with intact ventricular septum-is it safe after three weeks of age? Interact Cardiovasc Thorac Surg.2010;11(5):641-4.

[54] Huss JM, Kelly DP. Mitochondrial energy metabolism in heart failure: a question of balance. J Clin Invest 2005;115:547-55.

[55] Gupte RS, Vijay V, Marks B, Levine RJ, Sabbah HN, Wolin MS, et al. Upregulation of glucose-6-phosphate dehydrogenase and NAD(P)H oxidase activity increases oxidative stress in failing human heart. J Card Fail 2007;13: 497-506.

[56] Luzzato L, Battistuzzi G. Glucose-6-phosphate dehydrogenase. Adv Hum Genet 1985;14:217-329.

[57] Gupte SA, Levine RJ, Gupte RS, Young ME, Lionetti V, Labinskyy V, et al. Glucose-6-phosphate dehydrogenase-derived NADPH fuels superoxide production in the failing heart. J Mol Cell Cardiol 2006;41:340-9.

[58] Iemitsu M, Miyauchi T, Maeda S, Sakai S, Fujii N, Miyazaki H, et al. Cardiac hypertrophy by hypertension and exercise training exhibits different gene expression of enzymes in energy metabolism. Hypertens Res 2003;26:829-37.

[59] Bergmeyer HU, Bernt E. D-glucose determination with hexokinase and glucose-6-phosphate dehydrogenase. In: Bergmeyer HU, editor. Methods of Enzymatic Analysis. London: Academic Press; 1974, p. 1196-1201.

[60] Zimmer HG. Regulation of and intervention into the oxidative pentose phosphate pathway and adenine nucleotide metabolism in the heart. Mol Cell Biochem 1996;160:101-109.

[61] Matsui R, Xu S, Maitland KA, Hayes A, Leopold JA, Handy DE, et al. Glucose 6-phosphate dehydrogenase deficiency decreases the vascular response to angiotensin II. Circulation 2005;112:257-63.

[62] Gupte SA. Glucose-6-phosphate dehydrogenase: a novel therapeutic target in cardiovascular diseases. Curr Opin Invest Drugs 2008;9:993-1000.

[63] Hink U, Li H, Mollnau H, Oelze M, Matheis E, Hartmann M, et al. Mechanisms underlying endothelial dysfunction in diabetes mellitus. Circ Res 2001;88:E14-E22.

[64] Park J, Rho HK, Kim KH, Choe SS, Lee YS, Kim JB. Overexpression of glucose 6-phosphate dehydrogenase is associated with lipid dysregulation and insulin resistance in obesity. Moll Cell Biol 2005;25:5146-57.

[65] Serpillon S, Floyd BC, Gupte RS, George S, Kozicky M, Neito V, et al. Superoxide production by NAD(P)H oxidase and mitochondria is increased in genetically obese and hyperglycemic rat heart and aorta before the development of cardiac dysfunction. The role of glucose-6-phosphate dehydrogenase-derived NADPH. Am J Physiol Heart Circ Physiol 2009;297:H153-162.

[66] Recchia FA, McConnell PI, Bernstein RD, Vogel TR, Xu X, Hintze TH. Reduced nitric oxide production and altered myocardial metabolism during the decompensation of pacing-induced heart failure in the conscious dog. Circ Res 1998;83:969-79.

[67] Lopaschuk GD, Folmes CD, Stanley WC. Cardiac energy metabolism in obesity. Circ Res 2007;101:335-47.

[68] Miana LA, Assad RS, Abduch MC, Silva GJ, Nogueira AR, Aiello VD, Moreira LF. Reversible pulmonary trunk banding VIII: Intermittent overload causes harmless hypertrophy in adult goat. Ann Thorac Surg. 2013 Apr; 95(4):1422-8.

[69] Fávaro GA, Assad RS, Abduch MC, Silva GJ, Gomes GS, Andrade JL, Krieger JE, Moreira LF. Reversible pulmonary trunk banding: VII. Stress echocardiographic assessment of rapid ventricular hypertrophy in young goats. J Thorac Cardiovasc Surg. 2013 May;145(5):1345-1351.

[70] Apitz C, Honjo O, Humpl T, Li J, Assad RS, Cho MY, Hong J, Friedberg MK, Redington AN. Biventricular structural and functional responses to aortic constriction in a

rabbit model of chronic right ventricular pressure overload. J Thorac Cardiovasc Surg. 2012 Dec;144(6):1494-501.

[71] Apitz C, Honjo O, Friedberg MK, Assad RS, Van Arsdell G, Humpl T, Redington AN. Beneficial effects of vasopressors on right ventricular function in experimental acute right ventricular failure in a rabbit model. Thorac Cardiovasc Surg. 2012 Feb; 60(1):17-23.

[72] Friedberg MK, Cho MY, Li J, Assad RS, Sun M, Rohailla S, Honjo O, Apitz C, Redington AN. Adverse Biventricular Remodeling in Isolated Right Ventricular Hypertension Is Mediated by Increased Transforming Growth Factor-β1 Signaling and Is Abrogated by Angiotensin Receptor Blockade. Am J Respir Cell Mol Biol. 2013; 49(6): 1019-28

[73] Assad RS, Zamith MM, Silva MF, Thomaz PG, Miana LA, Guerra VC, Pedra CA, Marcial MB. A novel adjustable pulmonary artery banding system for hypoplastic left heart syndrome. Ann Thorac Surg. 2007 Dec;84(6):2081-4.

[74] Abduch MC, Assad RS, Aiello VD. Experimental ventricular pressure overload in young animals induces cardiomyocyte hypertrophy in addition to hyperplasia of contractile and noncontractile elements of the myocardium. J Thorac Cardiovasc Surg. 2009 Jun;137(6):1573.